RELIEVED BUT *Deceived*

Living Life After Abortion

SUSAN J. RIDLEY

Relieved But Deceived
Susan J. Ridley

Printed in the USA
Copyright © 2002 by Susan J. Ridley
Reprinted August 2019
Library of Congress Cataloging-in-Publication
Data ISBN 9781698181547

Contents

Dedication

This book is dedicated to my oldest granddaughter, Seneca, who believes that my life experiences have helped her stay on the right path, and insists that in this book "I tell it all."

And to my four precious daughters – Darnetta, Fonda, Shelly and Karmen, who so unselfishly and without any hesitation were willing to have a part of their private lives exposed in the pages of this book.

Why I Am Publishing This Book – Again

Giving is an essential and important part of stewardship, as we have a responsibility of managing everything God gives us for His glory. This includes such things as our time, our wealth, our talents and our gifts. When the first book was published in 2004, I did not understand that it was an assignment from God. I don't recall ever thinking that writing a book or becoming an author was a gift.

Little did I realize that my decision to write a book on "getting rid of unborn babies" would have such a strong message and profound impact on helping women to see the other side of abortions. Never did I imagine that men would have such an interest in the book as well. Could it be that men are affected by abortions also? Through the years, countless women have asked about the book. Invitations to seminars and workshops have been missed due to a lack of publication. Although I did not recognize this as God's assignment at first, through the years I became fully aware that I was not helping people with an unpublished book.

Well, let's just keep it real. I always have to tell it like it is. I acknowledge my disobedience in not publishing this book sooner. One thing about God—he will perfect that which concerns us, and He's always giving us grace. About three years ago, a friend of mine whom I had not talked to in a while, called me. She said, "Girl, I'm not taking another whipping from God about your book. I am supposed to help you. It's needed. So when do you want to meet?"

We got started and almost finished when another former friend of mine known as "procrastination" showed up. Along with it came the familiar spirit of "aborting" things, not completing, and moving on to something else. Oops,

I'm still overlooking various areas of my life. But by God's grace and my friend, we completed the book. I know this book must be published again as this message is never ending for the world and for generations to come.

Abortions are still happening. Generally, the two types of abortions done today are in-clinic abortions, and the abortion pill. But, no matter how you "get rid of unborn babies," there will always be another side of abortions that needs to be addressed. Some years ago I created a 12-step program for abortion healing. With more than 25 women attending, many of them felt that they didn't really need any help. They knew God had forgiven them, and He had; he's a forgiving God. But what they didn't realize was the aftermath, the residue that comes with abortions.

I encourage you, whether you have experienced an abortion, or you know a family member or friend who has, or if someone crosses your path, it would help to have this book in your hands. Make it a part of your library and stewardship through the power of giving as we reach out and encourage healing in others.

To God Be the Glory!

Introduction

It was the late 50s when I had my first abortion. I didn't experience the modern day conveniences that are available at the abortion facilities today. There was no pre-abortion counseling and no videotapes to help you understand the procedures that would eliminate your pregnancy.

As a matter of fact, having an abortion was a secret... and definitely a moral issue, and many considered it a sin.

How much easier it is for today's women to make that choice. It doesn't matter what grandma thinks; after all, it's legal so it couldn't be that wrong. How little stress there is today, knowing there are medical professionals whom you can depend on, not to mention the reports that support women's rights to abort. How helpful to have colorful brochures and pamphlets that offer instructions for pain, medication and proper healing. I can truthfully say I understand why the abortion facilities are full, and why women make that choice. I DID IT—and without any of the above-mentioned amenities.

Yet there is another pain that the brochures and pamphlets can't convey. It's the emotional trauma that takes root after the abortion. Sometimes it happens right after the abortion and is played off or pushed aside, and sometimes it happens years later. No matter how much advice or counseling one may receive beforehand, *this pain can only be felt afterwards; it can only be experienced after the abortion.*

That's why I've got to tell my story. I've got to tell women the real deal. My story is simple—it's not complicated. I just didn't know the truth at the time of my actions. I didn't know the truth about how the hidden effects of aborting babies had infiltrated my very soul.

After becoming a Christian I began ministering to women at various workshops, conferences and retreats. God began to heal me from my past, as well as countless others, as I candidly shared my life experiences with them. My story entailed such things as teen pregnancy, sexual and physical abuse, divorce, and many other matters.

However, one area that I never fully dealt with was the abortions I had. Having spoken both nationally and internationally, I realized that I was stuck in this one area of my life. *I didn't feel that my abortions were wrong; after all, they were a relief.* Also, being a Christian, I knew God was not pleased with my attitude concerning abortions, and that my ministry would be hindered if I did not get in touch with this issue.

You see, I was one of those women who felt as though there was no aftermath, no ill effects or no problems from having abortions. After all, I had certainly gone on with my life. The abortions were now behind me. Now I was a Christian, happily married to a jewel (Ralph), involved in church, had my own ministry... my life was successful. I had absolutely no clue that many of my behaviors and the decisions that I made were from the ill effects and emotional trauma that often results from having abortions.

Unfortunately, it took too many years for me to get fully in touch with this buried area of my life. It shouldn't have taken me 30 years or so to do it, but it did. However, once I began writing this book I had to face the pain and the truth about my abortions. Yes, I was **Relieved But Now Deceived. But God Has Redeemed The Time** and has given me an opportunity to share my story.

NO NEED TO BE DECEIVED ANYMORE!

If you've never had the personal experience of having an abortion but you know someone who has, please make sure they read this book.

If you've already had an abortion(s), hopefully this book will help you identify and cause you to get on the road to complete healing and whole-ness. Or perhaps you're already on the road and this book will give you added strength and courage.

If you are contemplating having an abortion, perhaps my story will help you see what I could not see.

Acknowledgments

There are countless numbers of people who have been significant in my life throughout my ministry. I could not have made it without their love and support. Many have contributed much to the development of my character, my ideas and my accomplishments. It impossible to name everyone who aided me, so please forgive me now if your name is not mentioned. I will, however, acknowledge those who have been instrumental in the writing of this book.

To the women who supported the first women's ministry that I was involved with, **The Sisters Club** and later **RAAH Christian Women's Ministry,** much thanks for letting me be real with you. You allowed my God-given gift of openness and transparency to come forth, thus bringing about healing to me and many others.

Germaine Copelend, author of *Prayers That Availeth Much*, thank you for your persistence in encouraging me to get the first book out, and for not giving up on me (because it took me so many years to complete it). Also, thank you for allowing me to use your editor, **Donna Walker.**

Many thanks to my long distance friend from Georgia, **Lillian Douglas**, who insisted that I get away and graciously opened up her home, along with her husband **Fred**, and provided me with a most enjoyable and stimulating atmosphere to think, write and complete the pages of my book.

Althea Adams, who with such a willing heart and belief in my book, began typing my first manuscript.

To **Mary Smith,** who very patiently deciphered through my sloppy handwriting and helped me to think through what I had to say.

To **Tracey Evans**, who so faithfully stuck with me as I rearranged, changed, cried and sighed as she diligently gave helpful suggestions and support as we completed the manuscript.

Emmanuel Adams, author of *Poor Butterfly*, who became my forerunner and encouraged me to move forward and publish my own book.

Dorothy Mitchell, long-time friend who has never grown weary in answering my many questions and helping me with various studies and research in the field of psychology and counseling.

Thanks to my sister-in-law, **Aretha Bryant**, and my friends, **Cereda Rispress** and **Pam Johnston**, thank you for being my cheerleaders. No matter what I was going through, or how much I complained or grew weary, you always reminded me of the former challenges that I had accomplished. You never let me forget the potential you saw within me.

Juliana Smith, thanks for your friendship,

your persistence and for being such a great resource person.

To the brother I never had but always wanted, **Danny Rispress.** You've always encouraged me by offering the right words at the right time.

To **Trevitt New Life Ministries,** my church family, thanks for your prayers and encouragement to hurry and get the book done, and to **Pastors' Bob** and **Odette Martin,** who showed so much patience and understanding as I fell short of my church obligations while completing this book.

To my mother-in-law, **Emma Ridley,** thanks for those ongoing words, "go to it girl." To my mother, **Pauline Johnson,** who had the challenging task of raising me as a single parent.

Thanks for passing on to me your outgo-ing personality and your organizational skills. They have been a tremendous help during this project.

To my five children and their mates:

Les (Son); and wife, Mary;
Darnetta (Daughter); and husband, Tim;
Fonda (Daughter); and husband, Kevin;
Shelly (Daughter); and husband, Bryan;
Karmen (Daughter), and husband, Tim.

You all believed in me so very much. You give me so much strength, hope, joy and encouragement. You're always pushing and promoting any project, goal or vision that I have. You all keep me alive.

To my husband, **Ralph Ridley,** you are the joy of my life! Thanks for loving me unconditionally and allowing me to be me. I appreciate your continued support, and how you never got tired of reading and re-reading, until we had a completed manuscript.

1
SECRETS

Be quiet now… Take not this matter to heart.
2 Samuel 13:20 (Amplified)

OH NO, NOT AGAIN!
IT COULDN'T BE…

And yet I knew that deep down within what I was anticipating was not going to happen, at least not for a while. My monthly cycle was one, one-and-a-half or two-months late. Perhaps it would be seven or eight more months before I would have it. It depended on how far along I was.

Surely this could not be happening to me

again. It was unfair. All of my girlfriends had sex much more than I did. Why was I the one who seemed to get caught?

There was a sick, empty feeling gnawing at the pit of my stomach, and tears that would not stop as I waited frantically from day to day for a show of blood. All the while wondering what people would say. THIS WAS ALL TOO FAMILIAR. This had happened before. It hadn't been that long ago that these same feelings had engulfed me.

It was actually just a couple of years ago when I was 14. My girlfriend kept telling me, "Oh, don't worry. You have a cold and that keeps you from having your period sometimes." I tried to believe her. I tried desperately to find something that would give me hope that I wasn't going to have a baby. Surely this was a nightmare. In the morning, I thought, I'd wake up and it would be all over. After all, I had only done it one time. My boyfriend had been trying to convince me to have sex and, of course, most of my girlfriends did it. So, eventually, I did it—in the back of the schoolyard.

I was leaning up against an incinerator, standing up, not even laying down. It was only a split-second. HOW COULD I BE PREGNANT? This was my first time. I had never, ever had sex before.

I will never forget that Saturday morning that I heard my mother and grandmother whispering from upstairs. I was doing my weekly chores. Being nervous, suspicious and afraid that they had discovered my secret, I hollered upstairs to them, "What are you two talking about?" I was not prepared for the words that followed as my grandmother said, "We were just wondering why all those clean Kotex are wrapped up in the trash can. There is nothing on them. And we also found a few of them that look like catsup has been spread on them."

Fear gripped my total being. They had discovered my secret; my whole body was numb. My heart was racing and my head was pounding from trying to hold back the tears. I tried to explain in a calm voice that it was nothing to be concerned about... I was late but I hadn't really done anything. But it was all over—they knew. I had to face the painful experience of being a little girl who was going to have a baby. The next few days were probably the saddest days for me. I wanted to run; I wanted to hide but there was nowhere to go. I felt so alone—so afraid, so confused. The tears were endless. It wasn't long ago that I was still a virgin.

Now I was going to have a baby. How did this happen? A friend had told me it (sex would feel good. Another friend said it would hurt at first because I was a virgin, and there would be blood. None of that happened. No good feeling; no pain; no blood. It seemed as though the right things had happened in order for me to be pregnant. As the days passed by, I began to think about an incident that had happened to me, one that I had tried to forget.

Several months prior to this, something

terrible happened. My boyfriend didn't know about it yet. Only one person knew about it, and that was my girlfriend. I made her promise to keep it a secret.

One evening while at Poindexter Recreation Center, I was talking with a guy whom I knew and who was a friend of my boyfriend. My boyfriend would not be at the recreation center until later, when he got off work (he had a part-time job). While we were chitchatting, he suggested we go play on the swings until my boyfriend arrived. Of course, this meant being out of the building and going around the back where the swings were. I had absolutely no hesitation at all; I completely trusted him. I never once thought about what would happen next. I don't recall getting on the swings.

The next few moments seemed like hours as I found myself fighting for my life. I remember fighting hard, really hard. He began to try and rape me, but I was kicking, hollering and frantically trying to convince him to stop. Suddenly he pulled out a knife. I don't recall if it was big or small but I know that at this point I quit fighting. I was terrified as he raped me up against a big building that was in back of the recreation center. Afterwards, he began to cry in a sick sort of way, and kept apologizing, saying that he was sorry. He didn't know I was a virgin.

I was very scared and confused. He also made me promise not to tell. He said if I did he would kill me because I knew he was watching as I walked into the center. My girlfriend and I started playing the piano. I was trying to laugh and act like we were having fun, but at the same time I was telling her what had just happened (I knew he was watching me).

We went to the girl's restroom and that's when we saw all the gravel and dirt in my clothes, and all over the lower parts of my body. Oh yes, and just like others had said, there was blood and the excruciating pain. It all happened during the rape. That's when my virginity was stolen.

I made my girlfriend promise not to tell. I just tried to forget the whole incident. That was a secret no one would ever know.

I knew that if I told my mother, I couldn't go to the recreation center again. If I told my boyfriend, I thought he would say it was my fault because I went willingly to the back of the center. I felt so empty and even dirty. I didn't know anyone who had been raped.

Remembering and re-thinking about this incident and secret gave me a clearer understanding of what had happened to my body. I really wasn't a virgin as I had thought during the time that my boyfriend and I were leaning up against the incinerator; not at all. My body had been ripped open by the rapist several months prior. This horrible and terrifying experience had left my body exposed and vulnerable.

Perhaps this was the answer I needed as to why it seemed that I got pregnant so easily with my boyfriend. Looking back, I am truly grateful that I didn't get pregnant by the rapist.

Getting pregnant at 14 and giving birth at 15 was finally behind me. NOW HERE I WAS AT 16, AND PREGNANT AGAIN FOR THE SECOND TIME!

2

MIXED MESSAGES

*Train up a child in the way he should go: and
when he is old, he will not depart from it.
Proverbs 22:6*

My second pregnancy was very different because my stepfather became my savior. He was able to convince my mother that I should not have this baby. I don't recall the word "abortion" ever being used, but he knew a prominent doctor who would help settle the matter.

My stepfather loved me very much, and I knew that he was doing what he thought was best. After all, I was so young, already a mother, and another child would certainly not help matters.

I also knew that abortion was not my mother's decision, and that she was being persuaded by my stepfather. She was paying a family (who were friends of our family) to keep my daughter (first child) while I finished high school. Surely we didn't need the hurt and humiliation of me having another child out of wedlock.

I was never asked any questions. I don't recall the time of year or the season, but I do know it was dark outside. I don't even have a vague memory of the doctor, the procedure, the room—nothing. But I knew that after I left the doctor's office I wasn't pregnant anymore, and it was all right. After all, my parents had to be right, and me not having another baby was surely a good choice. I had one child, I was doing well in school, and life needed to go on. Even then I felt a great sense of relief.

This decision made by my parents, the most

significant people in my life, would assuredly be beneficial to me. Or would it?

I believe that it was at this point, through this experience, that the root of death took hold in my life. Getting rid of babies became a way of life for me.

When significant people approve, give you permission or affirm you, their affirmation seems to make things right. I knew having sex and getting pregnant was not proper, but at least there was a solution. Just get rid of it. It must not be all that bad. After all, my parents must think its okay. Whether this was truly the way they felt or not, I don't know, but it was my perception of the matter.

Looking back now, it's amazing how scriptures, even though you may not be aware of them, can work in your life. I thought of Proverbs 22:6, *"Train up a child in the way he should go; and when he is old, he will not depart from it."* Here's an example of what I mean. When a child is trained up in an alcoholic family or an abusive home, often-times those patterns are imprinted into the child's soul.

While I could certainly not hold my parents responsible for my continued abortions, I believe that their decision to allow me to have an abortion became a pattern that took deep root. In spite of all the good and positive training my mother, grandmother and step-father directed towards me, the negative behavior became dominant.

Of course, as in most families, the matter of my having an abortion was never discussed. So no one really knew how anyone truly felt. I know now, after writing this book that my mother did not agree with my stepfather's decision so she blocked most of it out of her mind.

Uncomfortable subjects are often avoided when they should be addressed. No matter how old you become as parents, your adult children will look to you for approval or disapproval, acceptance or non-acceptance, opinions right or wrong. Although your children might argue with you, get angry or disagree, in the long run they want honest, legitimate answers.

Too often as parents we give mixed messages. As Christians, we say we believe the Word of God. We tell our children to live by the Word of God, but then we give them an opposing alternative. We give our permission, or even insist that they utilize birth control methods—yet never helping them to do what the Word of God says, "No premarital sex." What a mixed message! Don't have sex, but just in case you do, use protection.

While it may seem like logical advice, the message becomes confused and clear at the same time. Mom or Dad says one thing, but they really mean for me to do another. Isn't this a mixed message? It was for me, and I became culpable to choosing the convenient way out.

3

PATTERNS

For the good that I would do, I do not;
But the evil which I would not, that I do.
Romans 7:19

Over the next few years of my life, getting rid of babies became a pattern. If you notice I said, "getting rid of babies," rather than "having abortions." At this time, abortions were illegal and definitely a moral issue. It was looked down upon intensely, and it was certainly not a topic for open discussion. To do such a thing would label you as a person of low moral standing. It was definitely a secretive affair. You seldom heard the word discussed, yet you knew it happened. I knew of one incident in high school where a beautiful young girl died from having an abortion.

The word "abortion" had become popular in the '70s and '80s. Although women had experienced them for years, it had not yet been identified as a significant social concern. There were no abortion clinics around, and you certainly couldn't find them in the yellow pages.

The professional doctors who performed abortions were both undercover and expensive. You had to know someone to get a connection. Many "quacks" performed them as well. I experienced both types of abortion—the work of a professional and a quack.

No one helped me with the second abortion I had. Or should I say, no one made the choice **for me**. I convinced myself that a baby had no place in my life. I was probably 20 or 21.

By now I was divorced and had my hands full with two children. I'd recently experienced the death of one of my children who was only a year old. The last thing I needed was a baby.

Besides, this pregnancy was definitely a "slip up."

Again, another prominent doctor (not a quack) helped me out of my dilemma. Feeling compassion for me after hearing my sad story, he prepared me to miscarry. He reluctantly made my office examination a little more painful than usual.

Skillfully, he did what was necessary for me to go home and wait until the aborted miscarriage took place, so that I could then go to the hospital. I told myself, "This won't happen again. I'll get it together, but at least for now **"I'll just get rid of it!"** Once again, I was relieved of having a child.

The third abortion was not even a matter of thought or discussion. After all, who would want to be pregnant by a married man? Never mind the fact that he was much older, good looking, full of charm and made me feel special. You couldn't have told me that once he found

out I was pregnant he would ignore me
(like the plague).

Desperately, I confided in my girlfriend.
She had heard of a doctor in a small town in
Ohio who used to perform abortions. The
problem was she had no clue as to how we
could contact him since he was no longer
practicing medicine. Again, out of desper-
ation, I called information and asked for the
name of the doctor. Blood rushed to my
head and my heart was skipping beats as I
frantically waited and hoped that the right
person would answer the phone and free me
—once again—from another unwanted pregnancy.

Finally, a voice said, "Hello," and I said to
him, "I need help. Will you help me?"

With much anger and in a loud voice he
asked, "Who are you and how did you get
my number?" I told him that the operator
gave it to me. He said, "My number is
unlisted; you should not have been given
this number. I don't know you."

I don't really remember all that was said or how the conversation went after that. I only remember thinking, "Please don't hang up. Help me; please listen to me."

The next day my girlfriend and I took the day off from work at the Columbus Depot and she drove me to the address that he had given me over the phone.

There wasn't much pain or anything that was significant when the abortion was being performed. I don't remember the cost but out of my neediness, no cost would have been too much to set me free from having another baby.

After the procedure, while coming home, there was extreme bleeding that lasted several hours. But most of all was that feeling of relief—another baby that I didn't have to worry about.

By now, I'm sure you're starting to see the picture—the pattern. For me, the pattern that surfaced was, "If you're pregnant, **just get rid of it!**" I'm sure you're also starting to see the promiscuity that was also a part of my life. You're probably thinking, "Why didn't she use birth control? Why keep getting pregnant?" The best way I can explain it to you is that if you've never been there, you probably won't understand it.

Truthfully, having sex at that time was never really a big thing as far as pleasure or enjoyment was concerned. It was something that was more or less expected in a relationship or a date. It was just what you did to prove yourself to them.

Of course, there were those unexpected times when you tried so hard to convince yourself that you would no longer be sexually active, only to fall into the same trap again and again. After all, I was getting something in return for sex, too—money, acceptance, attention, fulfillment of lust, gifts for my children, new outfits, and lots more. What the heck!

I have yet to mention the waves of emotional trauma that brought about and feelings of guilt, shame, fear, depression, worthlessness, and low self-esteem. Time and time again I tried to get what I thought I needed by using my body as a vessel. However, each time I ended up with the same empty vessel. Beginning at age 14, when I became pregnant with my first child, and continuing through the age of 21, I had birthed three children. My high school graduation was marked with significant trauma. At the time I was three months pregnant, I had one child who died at one year of age, and there were three abortions in my history, for a total of six pregnancies.

You may find this next statement hard to believe but it's true. Every time I had sex without some form of birth control I became pregnant. At that time, my choice of birth control was having my partners use protection (rubbers). The pill caused me too many problems so I didn't always use it. I thank God that somehow, in this mixed-up part of my life, I didn't contract a venereal disease, or any real serious female problems.

God's protection was with me even then. Evidently, He knew my life would take a turn for the better.

Don't misunderstand my frankness. I was not thrilled by what was happening in my life concerning these pregnancies. Up to this time, the three abortions I'd had were all performed by doctors. Not that it really mattered; my heart had become somewhat callous toward having babies. My attitude was, "If I get pregnant **I'll just get rid of it!**" I was rapidly becoming a pro at getting rid of babies. However, the next abortion (number four) was quite different. It didn't happen by going into a nice doctor's office. It was not at all what I was expecting.

Allow me to sidestep a bit before going any further. I want to share something here that many Christians may not agree with. I didn't know it then but I know it now. *Even in my sin, I discovered that God's guiding hand was upon me.*

At this particular point, my life seemed to be taking a turn for the worse. I began to settle for less. You know how porterhouse steak and hamburger are both beef but one costs a lot more than the other? You know how hamburger is a lesser grade than the steak? That's how my life was beginning to go.

Up to this point my promiscuity was somewhat limited to men with whom I had an established relationship, even if it had been for a short time. I didn't go to bed with just anybody. However, I was starting to think a little differently now, and I was wondering what it would be like if I became a real call girl and made plenty of money. I'm not talking about a "street whore" (I would never do that), but something a bit more sophisticated.

Being totally naïve and just plain dumb, I got tricked by a man who promised to give me a leather coat in return for sex. I did not realize that this man was capable of seriously hurting me, and that he had no intention of giving me the coat that he had promised. All he wanted was my body.

What I did get in return for my ignorance was another pregnancy. This was one of those times that protection was not used. I knew I had gone too far; I didn't know anything about this man and I had a sick, scary feeling about my new predicament.

From this point I was aware that God was with me, even though I continued in sin. As I said, I know that many people would not agree with me that God was present with me in the next few years of my life. That's probably because I did not acknowledge Him as my Savior, but I knew He was there nonetheless.

As I pondered my new predicament, my mind tried desperately to figure out who would help me get rid of this baby. Remember, it was the '60s and abortion clinics were not around. I was now involved with a new man who was 10 years older than me. He was a man of the streets who sold drugs, gambled, pimped women, and so on. However, he became wholeheartedly interested in me.

When I told him I was pregnant by this man who had tricked me, he became furious. He wanted to hurt him (if not kill him). He had encountered previous dealings with this man and did not like him. I begged him not to do anything and he agreed, but only if I would get rid of the baby I was carrying.

Of course, nothing sounded sweeter to my ears than to get rid of the baby. My new male friend (I'll refer to him only as "friend") made the arrangements and took me to a house for the procedure. Like my other abortions, there was no pre-abortion counsel offered. I was told to get on a table. This was where I encountered my first coat hanger abortion.

Fear gripped me from my head to my toes. I remember very little as I was close to being petrified. There were only three people in the room: my friend, the abortion man and myself. Oh yes, and God had to be there with me, watching over me. I don't recall what it felt like totally, but I think I remember when the coat hanger ruptured the sac. Fear penetrated my very being, both emotionally and physically.

I wish the story could end here, but it doesn't. Somehow I was further along in my pregnancy than I had realized, and what should have happened with the coat hanger didn't work. I had lots of pain and bleeding, but no big blob ever came out. I was delirious for two days, with a temperature well above normal.

The abortion man said I must have been further along than he had expected. He said I needed to go to the hospital but I had to keep quiet about the procedure. Somehow it was agreed upon between him and my friend that he would try to puncture the sac again. I honestly don't remember where the next attempt took place. I just remember that several hours later, in my bedroom, a dead fetus, a little boy about four and a half to five months, came out of me. We put it in a plastic bag and threw it into the incinerator in back of the apartment where I lived.

You can't possibly tell me that God wasn't watching over me. Only His mercy can deliver you in time of great trouble. God allowed my friend to stay in my life for a few years. The reason I say that God allowed my friend in my life is because he settled me down. I wasn't running the streets and having men anymore. We became a couple and were true to one another.

Although my friend's street life never completely ended, he no longer had other women. He became employed and changed his lifestyle for me. We had a child together, a girl whom he adored for the very short time he was in her life. I was never really in love with him but was captured with his charm, his kindness, his tenderness, and the true love he had for me. But it was not meant for us to remain together. This sinner man had truly come into my life for a season and caused me to turn my life around from the road of destruction on which I was headed. Later I learned that he was a backslider who had known the Lord at one time, and I believe God used my friend to rescue me.

Please understand that I was still a sinner and doing wrong, but my promiscuous life took a turn for the better when I met my friend. We broke up when our daughter was about a year old. I heard years later that he was killed in California as he continued on with his previous lifestyle in the streets. Even without my serving God, a fool would recognize that God had spared my body and my life.

You would surely think that my declaration of no more abortions would be an easy decision to make for my life. However, when I became pregnant again, the fear did not override the need, and another abortion would ensue.

This would be abortion number five. This time, however, there was a new fear. Not just being afraid of a coat hanger penetrating my body, tearing and ripping it apart, or of mutilating a baby, but there were other fears as well. In rapid succession, these questions flooded my mind:

- What was becoming of me?
- Was I no longer conscious of right and wrong, of good and evil?
- What kind of person was I anyway?
- What if I died from this coat hanger or got an infection… what would happen to my children? Who would care for them?

Other questions infiltrated my mind such as:

- Who am I? What am I doing?
- Where is my mind? What are my goals?
- Where are my morals? Who am I hurting?
- What's happening to me?

The abortion took place on my girlfriend's table with her, the abortion man and myself present. She could hardly hold my legs apart; I was shaking like a washing machine that was off balance. One thing I knew for sure was **this would be the last one**. I didn't know what was becoming of my life but I knew that this was the last time I would get rid of a baby. I remember saying, "God help me; don't let me die! This is it; I've got to change." And God heard me; He didn't let me die. **HE STILL HAD A PLAN FOR MY LIFE!**

4

GOD HAD A PLAN
IN SPITE OF...

*And Jesus said unto her, neither do
I condemn thee; go, and sin no more.
John 8:11*

As I stated in the previous chapter, my life was taking a turn for the better. I began to focus on the wrong things I was doing. I knew that God had spared my life every time I had an abortion. I also knew I never wanted to experience getting rid of another unborn child again. I became dissatisfied with the way I talked to my children, always cussing and screaming. I yelled constantly and I knew that as far as providing for them was concerned, I was a good mother. We had lots of fun together and I took them places, but I just wasn't the mother I wanted to be. I wanted my kids to be involved in Sunday School, but I couldn't seem to get them to a church.

I still liked going out and partying, but honestly, many times it was an effort to prepare to go out, but I certainly didn't want to be square and miss the fun. After all, partying all night was the thing to do.

Meeting different guys was starting to get old. I realize now that thinking that I needed a man was just a standard set by society. Really, I enjoyed being with my children. I didn't want to appear odd, so I continued to have a male friend. After all, weren't you supposed to have a man, or at least be looking for one? Fortunately, if I chose to bring the men I dated around my children, they were always nice to them, and we often did things together.

I wasn't really looking for a husband. I had already been in an abusive situation when I was a teen. I got married at 18 to a guy I was dating since I was 16, and I was divorced at age 19. So, marriage really wasn't on my agenda. However, I was involved with an older man (what we called a "Sugar Daddy") who was perhaps 30 years or so older than me. He was married, so there was very few demands put on me in the relationship. I just got what I wanted materialistically and dated other men on the side. However, I wasn't happy. I cried a lot, and was also depressed. I wanted more out of life than working, dating and partying.

I was becoming more and more discontent with my life. I knew I needed something, but certainly not God. How could God, who was way up in heaven, somehow, possibly help me? Besides, my problems were my own; I would work them out. Funny, isn't it, how I would call on God in my troubled times yet I didn't want to serve him?

In the file room where I worked at the Columbus Depot, my co-worker (an old-school and neighborhood friend) was constantly telling me that I needed the Lord. She was trying to get back to God herself and she recognized that I needed him as well. She told me she was praying for me. Later on I found out that my grandmother's Sunday School class and other church people were praying for me.

Apparently, the prayers were beginning to work and my attitude began to change towards going to church. At this time, the simultaneous revivals were going on among the Baptist churches in my city. I only knew that because someone invited me to attend. I promised to go that Sunday. After all, I wanted my children to attend church, and years had passed since I had been.

Now please understand, going to church was not foreign to me. I attended a Pentecostal Church with my grandmother from the time I was born until I was 12 years old. However, I had never given my life to Christ.

From what little I could remember, my grandmother's church was really strict, so I didn't want to go there. We couldn't wear jewelry or make-up, so they looked a bit homely.

On Friday night, two days before the Sunday that I was to attend church, I went out as usual to the Macon Club. Little did I know that God was already at work in my heart. I started crying profusely when I arrived at the club for seemingly no reason at all. This was my partying time and there I was, sobbing as if someone had died. When my girlfriend and others asked me what was wrong all I could say was, "I don't know."

At that time, my favorite song was, "Ain't Nobody Home," and my favorite dance song was the "Philly Dog." Somehow, the song was getting on my nerves and I didn't want to dance. Crying seemed to be the only thing I could do. I went home confused and not understanding what was happening to me.

Saturday night I stayed home because I knew that on Sunday I would be going to church as I had promised. For me, to not go out on a Saturday night was a miracle. Could God be doing something? That Sunday was the turning point in my life.

I went to Refuge Baptist Church on 20th Street, which was down the street from the Macon Club. The guest preacher was talking about Job. Now anyone who went to Sunday School had heard about Job, but not me. This message hit me like a ton of bricks! I could not believe what Job went through. It was the greatest story I had ever heard, and I cried during the whole message.

I didn't know where my kids were, perhaps in a children's class or something, but the very next thing I knew, my children were going up the aisle to join church. Now I really began crying. Here my children were taking the step that I needed to take. That day, a true conversion took place in my life. I remember the people looking at me like they were telling me to turn to Jesus. You know church folk know when God's doing something in you, but I stayed in my seat crying.

I went home that Sunday and could hardly wait to get to work the next day. As stated earlier, I worked in the file room. It was a large area where lots of people sat at individual stations. We were like a family; we mingled, ate, had fun and, of course, worked.

On Mondays, some of us liked to come together and share what our weekend was like. I usually had something funny or some dirty gossip to share, and my stories always got attention. On this particular Monday I came in like a wild woman. I was telling them about Job and what had happened in his life. When I finally calmed down, I realized that some of my co-workers had frowns on their faces; others were laughing and some were staring at me as if I'd lost my mind. Some were absolutely astonished! No dirty jokes, no weekend experiences with men or partying, but all about God and what he did in Job's life.

Every night that week I went to the revival. On Monday I called my girlfriend and said, "Let's go to church." She said, "What? This is the night we go to the 502 Club on St. Clair Avenue. What is wrong with you?" Again, I started crying. I said, "I've got to go to church." She told me to go on but not with her that night.

My daughter, who was about to turn eight years old at this time said, "Mama, don't cry. I'll go to church with you." So we went in a cab to church.

On my job there were whispers and lots of doubt that this new thing that had taken hold of me would not last. Some men even made a bet that it would be over soon—our or five weeks at the most. Actually, it went out all over the depot that the little "fast girl in 306" got saved.

My life began to change immediately and I had a thousand questions. I barely did my work in the files. I spent most o my time talking with Christians and asking questions about their experiences. I was about to burst with joy! Everyone knew it; I could not hide the change. I still continued to cry in every church meeting, but I don't recall ever going up front to become a part of the church.

By now, my grandmother was telling me that I should join the church I was brought up in, and that I needed the Holy Ghost. She plainly let me know that, in her opinion, I was not saved. I needed more and I didn't have anything. I resented this very much because I did have something. I know she meant well but I knew I had changed.

In her Pentecostal church, you were not considered saved unless you were baptized in Jesus' name and spoke in tongues. So, from her point of view, I didn't have anything. I hadn't even been baptized and I certainly had not spoken in tongues, but I knew I had truly been converted. It wasn't so much that I resented what she believed, but the fact that she could so easily discredit my experience with God. Of course, this caused me to rebel against her (but not for long). I was so excited and hungry for God that I was willing to try whatever anyone said. Had my grandmother approached me in a more loving way, she would have easily persuaded me that God had even more for me to receive.

Several weeks later, on March 26, 1967, a husband and wife team came to my house and told me about receiving the Holy Ghost with evidence of speaking in tongues. They were my girlfriend's aunt and uncle, and she told them that I was crying all the time, and that I still had not joined a church. They also belonged to my grandmother's church.

That night I was baptized in water and spoke in tongues. I will *never* forget that experience. When I came home, my mother stared at me. She said I looked different. The joy and peace I experienced that night will always be one of the highlights of my Christian experience. Little did I know that God was setting things in order. He was already planning my life.

I became a member of the Church of Christ of Apostolic Faith in Columbus, Ohio. This was also my grandmother's church. I loved my new found friend, Jesus, and I was truly getting closer to him. My worldly interest quickly changed and I became very involved in church.

Approximately five months later, in the summer of 1967, I was at the Monday night young people's meeting. That night the Lord caused Ralph Ridley to open his eyes and see me. I was now 24 years old. Ralph had been saved since he was eight years old and had always served God. Ralph had been a devotional and youth leader. He was a young man who loved the Lord and everybody knew he was a Christian. He stood out like a shining light.

In the school assemblies, Ralph was the guy who led the prayers. Many of the mothers in the church hoped God would put Ralph together with their daughters. He was the kindest, most gentle man you could ever meet. And God had a plan...

The bible states, *"He who findeth a wife findeth a good thing (Proverbs 18:22)."* Can you imagine God looking at me, in spite of all the promiscuity and abortions I had, and caused a man, Ralph, who loved and served Him with all his heart and soul, to find me? Well, he did, and on March 16, 1968, a little less than one year from the night I got saved, I married Ralph Ridley. We had a big church wedding, something I never dreamed would happen to me.

Oh yeah, I forgot to tell you this part. Ralph was saving himself for his wife, so he had not given himself over to fornication. He was still a virgin and God, in spite of it all, cleaned me up, turned me around and made me a virgin, too. Ralph and I experienced sex or the first time on our wedding night. He married me with my three children, and we had two more.

Ralph adopted my three children, changing their names to Ridley. Together, we raised five children who are all married, and they have blessed us with 17 grandchildren and 20 great-grandchildren so far.

In March 2018, we celebrated our 50th year of marriage. We have been in ministry together since we were married. This was also Ralph's desire, that God would send him a wife who loved reaching out to the lost and unsaved. Our hearts have always been knitted together as we have done extensive outreach ministry.

In the '80s, we had a halfway house for women who had fallen through the cracks of life and needed a helping hand. It closed in 1990 for lack of funds. We also served as part of a pastoral team in a local inner-city church in Columbus, Ohio.

Many years have passed as I recommission this book. I started writing it in late 1990. At present, I have a fruitful and full life. Much good has been accomplished, but obviously, I have other purposes to fulfill. Even though it took me many years to get to the root of my problems, my story would still be incomplete without dealing with the abortions.

5

DIGGING UP THE ROOTS

Behold, thou desireth truth in the inward
parts; and in the hidden part thou
shalt make me to know wisdom.
Psalms 51:6

As long as I was a sinner without the spirit of God, I didn't have to face the truth. I could cover up my mess and pain by being the party girl, having fun, being promiscuous and continuing with addictive behaviors, or by helping others (somebody was always worse off than me). But now I had become a sure enough, born-again tongue-talking Christian, and God wasn't giving me any slack. He started pulling the covers off of me immediately.

Doesn't the Bible also say that, "We reap what we sow?" As a matter of fact, God didn't show me all the junk that was in me until I got saved. I had to face certain areas of my life head-on that had been hindering me. Although I was not fully aware of what God was doing, He wanted to eventually use me mightily in deliverance ministry. He wanted me to help others out of their pain and traumatic experiences, and to encourage them to move on in the things of Him. God waited until I got saved and said that I wanted truth in my inward parts before he began to deal with my past issues.

These issues, inclusive of such things as sexual abuse, an absentee father (my dad died when I was two and a half years old, leaving my mother a widow with me to raise), low self-worth, feelings of fear, guilt, shame, getting pregnant at 14, rejection, addictions, disappointments, divorce at an early age, and seeking male approval to fill my emptiness, was manifested in my now saved, sanctified life.

No longer could I hide my unresolved past in worldly ways. God was saying I should be made whole—spirit, soul and body.

At this time I didn't realize God was calling me specifically to deal with my inner man. I recognized that there was a deep desire in me to go deep within myself. For example, if my finger was hurting I wasn't satisfied with just having it stop hurting. I wanted to go deeper. Why was it hurting? What went wrong?

Actually, it was in the 1970s, shortly after I got saved, that God had called me to leadership, that is, "up front ministry." I was the chairman of a church club of young women called the "Sister's Group." I'd share things about "life's experiences," not knowing it was bringing about healing to many. Truthfully, some people told me I talked too much, and that I shouldn't tell all my business. I remember thinking before I'd go to the meetings that, "This time I'm going to keep my mouth shut," but it never happened. And people were helped as a result of my openness and honesty.

It was in the late 1980s that I became aware that God was using me to help others from within, but He had begun with allowing me to see myself first. During this time you didn't hear much, if anything, over the pulpit about the things God was having me to share. The late Dr. Evelyn Carter Spencer, affectionately known as Rev. Ev, was the first person whom I have ever heard talk from the pulpit as an evangelist at women's meetings on sexual abuse and soul ties. I am certainly not trying to minimize the many people who have written books and have taught on inner healing, but remember that inner healing was and still is a very controversial subject. During the 1990s many people started teaching messages that dealt with the soul and the inner person.

As an evangelist and teacher, I attended numerous conferences and meetings teaching women to deal with their hurts and painful experiences from the past. God had gifted me with the freedom and ability to disclose my own personal experiences. As I shared, whether through humor or tears, many lives were transformed, healed, and restored by God's power.

Even though I would teach on grief and forgiveness (which are two necessary factors in dealing with abortions), I didn't exactly believe what I was saying. It wasn't from the heart. The words coming out of my mouth didn't match how I really felt inside, or what I actually wanted to say when discussing abortions. But, after all, I was the speaker of the hour, a godly woman at that, and surely I had to agree with the Bible and the Christian view on abortions.

In the early '80s my husband and I had an outreach center where we offered seminars on various topics. On a couple of occasions we had Christian films shown on abortions. They were very graphic with an emphasis on discouraging abortions, because they displeased God. Even then, I couldn't really express how I felt inside. How could a person who loved and obeyed God as much as I did be so off in their view on abortions? You see, I didn't really think abortions were wrong; I saw them as a RELIEF for me.

Also, something else was happening on the inside. I was beginning to feel like a hypocrite. Even people who didn't confess Christ could agree that abortions were wrong. Even some people who had low moral standards could say they believed abortion wasn't right. I continued to cry out to the Lord, "Help me to get to the root of this problem!" I'd sought counseling on dealing with abortion. The counselor seemed very surprised that I could talk about my abortions with absolutely no sadness or remorse. I went on for three or four occasions and I finally cried some during one of the sessions.

The counselor was trying to help me identify the feelings one should have in my situation. After all, I had destroyed life. Where was the sadness, the sorrow or the repentance? I even remember her telling me that I needed to say goodbye to the children I had aborted, and that I would see them someday in heaven. My reply was, "I don't care about those babies. I didn't know them and I sure didn't want to see them in heaven."

At various times I would talk with someone concerning my abortions, looking for an answer that would help me to see how wrong my thinking was. Once, when talking to my dear friend and mother in the gospel, Rev. Ev, she said, "You have buried it so deep, it needs to be dealt with."

In the early '90s, I went to an inner healing workshop with the intention of finally dealing with my abortions. The healing process was wonderful; however, it did not include the abortions. I ended up getting in touch with another buried area in my life. It was concerning the death of my son who died when he was a year old. At this workshop, I said goodbye to the little boy whom I had loved so desperately and wanted to know and raise. His name was Marlon; he was the baby that I didn't think about getting rid of. He was conceived during the short time I was married as a teen. The other two children before him were born out of wedlock. There was, of course, guilt and shame that I carried, especially being so young. Somehow, I thought that having a baby while married would make me a "good person," so to speak. To get rid of this baby was not even a consideration. I had finally done something right.

Several months before attending this workshop some friends and I were talking. They asked me this question, "How did I deal with death, and had anyone close to me ever died?" I replied, "Oh, I handle death okay. My grandfather died but we weren't close." My friend looked at me in disbelief. One of them said to me, "Okay, you avoid going to funerals, but what about your son? You had a child who died."

I was stunned! How could I forget about my son, a darling little boy who was full of life and had a bright smile and outgoing personality? He had died of the croup when I was about 20 years old. I had completely pushed his death some place deep within.

How embarrassed I felt. I was aware of the fact that he had died and I had told others, but somehow I didn't seem to be in touch with it. ANYTHING UNRESOLVED WILL COME BACK AGAIN! Something will trigger it.

My friend's words were true. I avoided funerals as much as I could, and I dreaded being around the families and friends when death occurred. I never knew what to say. I felt so helpless; sometimes I'd be crying more than the families. I was definitely not the person to serve others during death.

I had retained no memory of my son's funeral. My mother told me about it, but even today, I can't recall what went on. However, being able to get in touch with those deep, buried feelings of his death and saying how much I loved him, and also saying goodbye to him has freed me from within.

Now I look at death differently. I have gone to several funerals alone, and, thank God, I am healing in this area.

I was indeed glad for this healing; however, I remember leaving the workshop feeling somewhat disappointed because, again, this searching issue was not settled.

Please understand I didn't feel guilty or shame because of the abortions. That was the problem. I couldn't identify what I felt other than RELIEVED! I knew it was not resolved within me; it was unsettled.

I began to do what many people do. I began to rationalize my concerns and I decided that maybe I was carrying this thing too far.

After all, God was using me mightily in the ministry. Perhaps the enemy was torturing me with this, and God had forgiven me.

AFTER ALL, I'VE BEEN FORGIVEN! NO NEED TO LOOK BACK. Through the years, I'd sought various methods of help, trying hard to be certain that the abortions in my life had been dealt with.

Having somewhat of a counseling background, I knew the importance of freedom from within, and I was more than ready to get in touch with my abortion issues. So why hadn't it happened?

The next step that I took was quite easy. I did as many Christians do. I decided that apparently when I got saved, God had forgiven me for having had abortions along with all the abortions. I was free!

No one needs to look back. 2 Corinthians 5:17 says, *"Old things are passed away, behold, all things become new."* Now that statement is absolutely true—God had forgiven me of my sins, but that had nothing to do with the effects the abortions had on my life.

Thank God, in spite of how I tried to convince myself that I was okay, the Holy Spirit kept on nudging me and causing me to realize that **you're not healed** in that area. Things just kept showing up.

Again, I strongly believe that anything in your life that is unresolved will come up again somewhere in your life.

If there are issues that have not been settled from within they will eventually be triggered, even if it takes years to do so.

Some of the ways that I knew **my abortion issues were not resolved or settled from within** were through my actions and behaviors:

- First of all, a little anger would rise up in me when the word "abortion" was mentioned, whether it was on TV, a news article, or whatever. Most of the time I could control the anger, so if others were present they could not detect it.

- I took care to avoid any discussions about abortions. Because of my honesty and openness, I knew that if I opened my mouth, the truth would come out about how I really felt. You see, I had that old mixed message, "You shouldn't have an abortion." And on the other hand, "Get rid of it, if that's what you want to do."

- Whenever I would see people carrying signs in front of any abortion clinics saying, "Don't Kill the Unborn Child," or "Save the Babies," I would feel a slow burn of anger rising within, and I would say, "Who do they think they are? Are they gonna help raise the kid?"

In the late '80s, in a meeting with some Christian sisters, one expressed the fact that she might be pregnant. Before I knew it I said, "Oh no, honey, you don't need a baby in your 40s. I'll go with you to the abortion clinic." Some of the women looked shocked.

After all, this was a Christian gathering. As for me, I justified her thinking by her age, the fact that she had grown children and that she did not really need a baby for her mental state. But deep down inside me the feeling was, "If you don't want a baby, don't have one. Get rid of it!"

My four adult daughters and I have very open and direct conversations concerning any subject. On several occasions, they have been very direct in asking me what I thought about abortion. Being a good Christian mom and wanting my children to do right, I would say, "You know your Dad's and my view on abortion. What does the Bible say?"

Finally, one day my daughter said, "Mom, I want a direct answer on how you feel about having an abortion." Suddenly I felt trapped —what do I say next? If this girl really knew how I felt, she would faint. I really don't remember what I told her but it wasn't the whole truth.

Without any doubt in my mind, I knew that I must get to the **root of my problem.** Even though I couldn't put my finger on it exactly, I realized that somehow, someway, I was still being affected by the abortions I had.

I knew that part of the traumatic experience was locked in my emotions, but what was it? I wanted to help generations of women avoid what I felt, but I could only go so far. I couldn't even consider taking anyone beyond the place where I was, and I was stuck.

It was late November 1996, after Thanksgiving, and I was lying in bed talking to God. I was telling Him how miserable my body felt. My legs and feet seemed to be getting weaker and weaker. Lately, it seemed as though the amount of weight I was carrying caused me to need more rest breaks during the day. I was used to a high energy level of activity and rest breaks were new for me. I was saying to God, "What is this? Why can't I get on top of this weight problem?" It seemed as though I could help the whole world with their problems, but I couldn't get on top of my own. That's when I heard the word **"self-hatred."** I rose up in the bed and exclaimed, "Oh, come on, God! That's a strong word."

As I laid there in His presence, he showed me myself. I began to see how I was slowly killing myself by eating. It was like a slow suicide. I was not taking the proper care of my body and had exploded into an excess of 87 pounds.

My body that had once been 135 pounds was now at its peak of 222 pounds! I have a small frame so my body was beginning to respond in negative ways to the added weight. Oh, I had no blood pressure or diabetic problems, only the pain from carrying the excess baggage. Not only the physical weight, but the emotional baggage as well. I didn't just eat, eat and eat.

There were many days that I didn't eat very much at all, but the problem was that I was punishing my body. I could not discipline myself to eat right and proper foods so that I could lose weight. I understood that discipline was a trait I lacked, and that it was a weakness in me that I needed to work on. Believe me, I'd been through all the major exercise and diet programs. I was not completely ignorant in this area. I had even dealt with the emotional and childhood issues that concerned overeating. However,

I knew that I wasn't free. Suddenly, the thought occurred to me that I was destroying myself, little by little. If I loved myself, *why was I slowly killing myself?*

The word "self-hatred" resurfaced and caused me to think a bit harder about it. What did it mean? What was the root cause? Could there be such an unresolved inward hatred in me that it was now showing up in the form of self-destruction? Now I could see that my eating was also a form of self-destruction. I didn't come right out and say to myself, "Let me self-destruct myself or destroy myself by choosing inappropriate eating habits," but my actions said it all.

In my messages to others, I would often express that if food made you drunk, I would be an alcoholic. I realized that my food addition was no different than any other driving force—alcohol, drugs, sex, gambling, or shopping. After all, I was aware of the various changes going on in my body, and I was not doing anything about them. So, was improper eating and not taking care of my body a form of hating myself? Was I really destroying myself with food? The questions continued, but there were no answers in view.

6

STOP PLAYING GOD!

*There is a way that seemeth right unto
a man, but the end thereof are the
ways of death. Proverbs 16:25*

On Thursday, December 5, 1996, I went to see my counselor. Thank God I did. It was one of the most rewarding days of my life. As I began to disclose and expose my feelings, it didn't take long for us (me and my counselor) to get to the point. The real issue surfaced that day.

Actually, I didn't really plan to talk about *abortion* at this session. I was there because of the word "self-hatred." I wanted to see how and where it might fit into my life. But God knows the true heart, and I surely had asked Him to help me.

Once again, He heard my plea. Contrary to what I thought I was there for, I began immediately to talk about the abortions. I realized once again there was no remorse, no shame, no sorrow or no sadness related to my actions. As I went over some of the gory details about the abortions, I soon noticed that my counselor was teary-eyed and her face was saddened. She was feeling what I could not seem to feel for myself.

My thoughts were racing in my mind. What had I done that was so wrong? It was just a big blob that I got rid of! Why couldn't I cry? In a very tender tone, my counselor said to me, "Susan, those were lives that you destroyed. When the egg and sperm united it became life. Regardless to whom, when, or whatever the situation, God creates life."

I quickly retaliated, "But you don't understand, it *was* a relief! It was a wonderful feeling of freedom. It was so convenient.

Those babies would have been in my way. I didn't feel sad, and I didn't feel bad. I felt relief, relief, relief."

She said, "Okay, maybe you couldn't feel sad, so don't worry about the feelings right now. But you have got to stop playing God. You need to ask for His forgiveness."

Wow, did her words hit home! I was always tell-ing people, "Stop playing God!" Could this be me? "What do you mean, 'Stop playing God?'" I asked. Her response penetrated my very soul. "You stood in God's place and you made the choice of deciding whether or not what He had created should live or die. You played God. Those were babies. Susan, you didn't just get rid of babies, you killed them, and that was murder," she said.

I would say, "get rid of it," or "just get rid of the big blob," because somehow saying "it" or "blob" didn't sound as harsh or as cold as saying "babies." I didn't like the word *"killed."* It didn't sound the same as *"get rid* of it." It seemed to be a much stronger word. And I was not a *murderer*, or was I?

I continued to worry with my thoughts. Perhaps I did have a "murdering spirit." Well, what was a murdering spirit anyway? I was very uncomfortable with these words. It seemed as though words were running around in my head, and they all somehow connected, but I didn't know exactly how.

Self-hatred, self-destruction, murdering spirit, murder, kill, get rid of… That night as I was lying in bed, I began to think about these words. "Self-hatred" was the first word that came to mind. Now it seemed as though all of these words were centered around my life. I knew I was getting close to something, but what? I knew that somehow God was answering my prayers, and that I wanted to be free within.

I also knew that He could only reveal to me as much as I would allow Him to, because He never goes against our will. So I continued to pray, "God, show me what I need to know. Don't let me shut down." The easy way out would have been to say, "God knows my heart, and if He wanted to reveal something about my past, He would." But I didn't go that route.

In the Bible, the Apostle Paul said, *"Forgetting those things behind... I press toward the mark* (Phil. 3:13-14)." We conveniently use scriptures for what we want.

But I had been with the Lord long enough to know that He wanted me to be whole in this area of my life. God was choosing to heal me of abortions through a simple step-by-step process, and like it or not, I was going to have to deal with it.

Today we want everything quick, fast, and in a hurry. Unfortunately, one of the reasons there are so many inner problems in the body of Christ is because for years the church didn't put much emphasis on the soul or the mind. They just tucked those things away, covered them up, kept hidden secrets, and wore a mask. But God was truly taking me another way. You see, God doesn't put words or thoughts in your spirit and you just ignore them.

I knew that these painful words were a part of my deliverance. I needed a clearer understanding of what those words meant, not just a dictionary definition of them. So I began to pray and ask God to totally reveal everything to me. I searched for materials on the words that were bothering me.

Actually, as Christians, this is the way we should approach the Word of God. Whatever God reveals to us, we should begin to diligently seek Him and search the Bible and other biblical materials to gain more insight. When God wakes us up with a word, or gives us a particular scripture, it is up to us to study, dig, and search it out so that we will get the full revelation of it.

If a medical doctor gives us a diagnosis, we want all the information we can find about it. As a matter of fact, we'll go to another doctor to get a second opinion, or we'll get information at the library and read medical books to get more insight on the problem.

We must begin to take care of our minds (soul) the same way. God wants us to be free from the things that bind us, but it requires some effort on our part.

I couldn't seem to shut out the words, *"Stop playing God!"* They were so clear; it was as though they were illuminated in my mind. I cannot tell you how many times in counseling sessions I had told others the same thing, "Stop playing God." Now here were these same words being directed at me. Strange, isn't it, how we can see someone else's stuff, but not our own? I couldn't help remembering how uncomfortable the session was becoming as the truth was being spoken. I was feeling quite uneasy.

It is a natural tendency to shut down or remove yourself (in your mind) when things are hitting home. Sometimes when people don't want to deal with something, they physically run out of the room. But as uncomfortable and uneasy as

I felt, I had great anticipation. I knew God was in control—I knew my freedom was on the way. It was true! I HAD TAKEN LIFE IN MY OWN HANDS! As I drove home from the counseling session that day, I could hear myself loud and clear *as when I had made the choice each time to get rid of my baby.*

My thoughts were:

- "Oh, this one would really be in my way. I'm too young to be tied down with a bunch of kids. Besides, this was a mistake anyhow. He's married, too. No—definitely got to get rid of this one."

- "Oh, I've been down this road before. I ain't hardly getting hooked up with that crazy, no good man again and I sure ain't having his baby."

- "Oh no, I don't believe I'm pregnant. Whatever I got to do, I got to do. Whatever it takes, having a kid is out of the question."

- "I must have been out of my mind—I don't

know how I messed up. I can't have a kid interfering with my life right now. No more babies for me."

While continuing to drive, I realized something. I still had no feelings of sadness, sorrow or remorse for what I had done. I just felt relieved. **But for the first time**, I realized that I had destroyed life. I could no longer say I got rid of it, or it really wasn't a baby, just a blob. I had to admit to my God (and to myself) that having abortions killed my babies. **Yes, I had to call it what it was**.

Finally, something broke within me. The tears began to flow like a dam had broken loose. I truly repented and asked God to forgive me for "Playing God." No matter how relieved I felt, or whether I felt anything at all, it did not matter. I knew that I had played God by deciding whether a baby should live or die, and that having abortions had stopped life. Oh, can you see the picture? Yes, I was relieved, but oh, how deceived!

It was on this same day in 1996, still driving home from my counseling session and thanking God for unlocking another door within me, that I heard Him say, **"This is your first book."**

7

CALL IT WHAT IT IS

And ye shall know the truth,
and the truth shall set you free.
John 8:32

Before you can be healed of anything, you must first get in touch with what it is. You must name it and then ask God to help, heal, and forgive you. For years I couldn't find my way out of denial and call the sin in my life what it really was. When you are not honest with what you do, you deceive yourself and hinder the healing process.

You have heard the saying, "An ace is an ace; a spade is a spade." So it is with sin. Sin has a name—lust is lust, lying is lying, murder is murder, adultery is adultery, and stealing is stealing. I hated the very thought of referring to myself as a murderer. I wouldn't murder a baby. People who do that type of thing are despicable.

I had begun to look at what I had done in another way. Just because I hadn't used a gun or a knife to kill someone physically didn't mean I wasn't guilty. I had allowed a procedure to take place through me that would terminate a life. I'd kept a baby from being born. Finally, I was beginning to gain some understanding of the matter. The mindset I had lived with since my first abortion as a teenager had become deeply rooted within me.

The words, **"just get rid of it"** were embedded in my spirit. When I became pregnant, the thought **"just get rid of it,"** was automatically triggered within me. I didn't realize it at the time but getting rid of babies had become another form of birth control. As long as I used the pill or a contraceptive, it kept life from taking place. If I got rid of it, it took away a life that had begun.

To get rid of it was just a modest way of saying, "just kill the baby." In general, murder means *"to kill, to do away with, to put an end to, or get rid of."*

Owning up to the fact that I had murdered these babies by allowing a procedure to *"kill, get rid of, or do away with them"* gave me additional knowledge to receive the freedom I needed by just admitting it.

The Truth Will Make You Free

Still, I needed clarity to the confusion that was running wild in my head—self-hatred, self-destruction, murdering spirit. Where did they all fit in? As I began to mull over my life and the paths I had chosen, I could see certain behaviors and patterns that were centered around getting rid of, doing away with, and killing.

In 1990 I attended my 30-year class reunion

dinner with the thought that I had enjoyed high school. As the class reminisced over the exciting events and incidents that had taken place, I realized that it was a very unhappy and unfulfilling time of my life. I felt very uncomfortable and not really a part of anything they were laughing and talking about. Upon leaving, I felt sad and different, like I didn't belong there. High school was miserable. Oh, don't get me wrong, I had girlfriends, and guys liked me. I was outgoing, laughed, and had fun, but the inside didn't match the outside. I dropped out of high school during the latter part of the 10th grade to have my baby.

When I returned to school to complete the 11th grade, things were different, such as:
— I wasn't the same after having a baby. I didn't feel as though I was good enough.
— I couldn't get rid of the negative thoughts and ideas that I could ever succeed in school. I just sort of gave up, feeling hopeless.
— There were not a lot of girls who already had babies, so I felt different (much less than the

other girls).

— I wasn't active or involved in any school activities. I remember how much I really wanted to be a part of the drama club. Really, deep down inside, I liked the stage, especially talent shows and my piano recitals from when I was younger.

— In my own eyes, I was a failure and wasn't doing any of the things I had wanted to do such as cheerleader, drama, school choir, or band. Nothing.

— I had no desire to make good grades; just passing was now good enough. Any thoughts of going to college were quickly annihilated.

In my mind, I settled that I was a *fast girl*. Actually, I really wasn't fast. Most of my friends were having sex, but they hadn't had babies and they were still active in school.

There were other things, however, that happened as well to help me believe that I was fast. One was that because I had a baby, people labeled me as fast.

Some of the moms really didn't want their

daughters hanging with girls who had babies, and the guys now thought I was easy prey.

Two incidents happened where teen boys whom I trusted and had grown up with tried to have sex with me, and I knew it was only because I had a child.

Also, while I was still a virgin, my step-father had always referred to me as fast because I wanted to go to dances and have fun. So it was easy for me to settle for being *fast*. After all, didn't I fit the description?

Another challenge to my life was my boyfriend. No, this was not the boyfriend I had my first child by.

Sometimes when I should have been at school I was with him. He had dropped out of school, so many of the things I did were not school related. In my heart, I wanted to be a good student, popular at school and involved in school activity. Back then, I didn't know that I was smart, bright and intelligent, and I did not realize my leadership qualities.

Fortunately for me, my mother, stepfather or grandmother never gave up on me. Neither did they discourage me when it came to making good grades and finishing high school. But no one really knew that deep down inside I really didn't feel good about myself. I cried a lot and learned to cover up my feelings. It was really difficult to pass from the 11th to the 12th grade, but I did it.

It was somewhere within this timeframe that the first abortion had taken place. I felt as though I was dying on the inside. Somehow, by the grace of God, I made it through high school. To be able to walk across the stage at my high school graduation, being 3 months pregnant by my boyfriend, killed every goal and ambition within me. This was my third pregnancy, and this wasn't how I'd planned my life. I wanted to go away to college and live in a dorm. I had pictured having all these "sisters" in college. My vision for success was shattered.

I felt really bad because I didn't have any accomplishments listed under my picture in the yearbook. I HATED MYSELF AND I HATED WHAT I WAS DOING. I'D FAILED MYSELF AND I'D FAILED MY FAMILY.

Self-hatred had taken root in me. I didn't know that what I felt was **shame** and **guilt.** I was very sad and lonely. That *murderous spirit* (doing away with) was in full effect. *A part of who I really was and wanted to be was slowly dying.*

My dreams, goals, and plans had been done away with. I had messed up. I had one baby, one abortion and was pregnant again, and I hadn't turned 18 yet. By now (1960, the year I graduated), several girls in the neighborhood were pregnant. Together we talked, shared our hurts and pains, and cried a whole lot. Actually, we had our own little support group, we just didn't know it. At least we understood what each other was going through. These weren't my college sisters but they sure were what I needed at the time.

Unless you've been there, it's hard to understand the pain of teen pregnancy. It's hard to watch all of your goals and plans go down the drain.

Fortunately, the mom of one of the girlfriend's encouraged and helped us to realize that having a baby wasn't the end of the world. She brought each of us an application from the Columbus Depot to take a test to become a clerk typist. It somehow gave me hope again, because I could type, and perhaps I could pass the test.

There were several months of waiting for test scores and the time of hiring. Even with this ray of hope, there was yet another huge stumbling block in my way. Their names were **shame** and **guilt**. They had taken a much deeper root than I had imagined, and they were fast becoming my best friends.

My life was all messed up. I felt so humiliated

and embarrassed by my life. It now consisted of two babies and one abortion. I what I had put my mom and grandmother through. Also, having my first baby caused a slight separation between my mother and stepfather. I was under a lot of pressure from my boyfriend to get married. However, he was not what I thought I wanted in a man. But at only 18, what did I know about a man?

My boyfriend was nice looking, built right, a sharp dresser, smelled good and had a cute smile and all of that, plus he was a womanizer. He was also very mean, controlling and abusive. He hit me on several occasions, cursed me out, and always called me names. Somehow, I thought his obsessiveness and jealousy were signs that he loved me.

Whatever he told me, I would settle for, even if I didn't agree with it. His excuse for not wanting me to be with my girlfriends (like going to a shower or wedding, etc.) never really made sense to me, but it would somehow keep me from going. If I did go, I paid for it later by a push, jerk or slap from him, and definitely a good cursing out.

Since he didn't really beat me bad during this time (like giving me a black eye or a show of blood), I didn't quite think of it as a *real* problem. Besides, after each such episode, he would tenderly and lovingly assure me that he was sorry, and that he really loved me, but I had caused him to have to handle things the way he did. He just wanted the best for us.

If I would just act right, he wouldn't have to hurt me or get angry. No matter what happened, I always ended up saying *I* was sorry.

Personally, when I was growing up as a child, I had not experienced any type of abuse or name-calling. My mother and grandmother raised me, and I had never even heard my mother argue with a man. When she married my stepfather, they had disagreements but never fighting or name-calling. So this was a whole new thing for me. Even though I didn't exactly know what love was, somehow I just wasn't convinced that the treatment I received from my boyfriend was the kind of love I wanted. But, what the heck! I had two babies (one was his) and besides, I did love him and he would change once we were married (or so I thought).

With all this confusion going on inside me, the good thing was that I had passed the typing test and was hired at the Columbus Depot. I have no words to express how it felt to be dressed up at 18, and going to a job as a typist. I felt like I was walking on the clouds. For me, I was now somebody. I had a job, a good paying job. Besides, I was young, cute, loved to dress and I could go on with my life. I loved people, fun and good times. And most of all, I could really be a good mom to my children. *Unfortunately, I did not stick with that plan.*

My mother and grandmother did not think that marriage at this point was what I should do. As a matter of fact, they were against it.

Besides, my life had taken a turn for the best. They were very supportive and I felt I could definitely make it. But the feelings of failure were ever present. I was still trying to make up for the things I did wrong. As least if I got married, I would be doing something morally right. My children would have a father, we would get a home with a fenced-in yard, and we would be a family. After all, the problems that we had would work themselves out, especially after we got married.

Although I didn't say such words to myself as self-destruct or self-hatred, my behaviors spoke loud and clear. I know now that I hated myself for my failures. When you hate yourself, you try to do things to make yourself feel better. You also subconsciously punish yourself for the things you did wrong.

Deep down inside I knew that getting married was not the solution. I was miserable just thinking about it, but on the other hand, it would make me feel like a better person. Marriage was accepted and right.

It's sad that I couldn't just accept my new job and move on to the next step. The door had already opened and all I had to do was go through it. I had survived and was now on the other side. I already had the strength and courage to go on. Instead of moving forward I reached back within myself, still trying to fix things, and went through a door that I felt I had to go through.

The marriage only lasted one year. I could not survive the name-calling, hollering, punches, kicks, slaps, blood, and all the things that go with abuse. The murderous spirit really became alive in me. I began to plan and plot just how I would kill this man. There was not a day that went by that I didn't think about how to get out of this situation. To kill him before he killed me was becoming a thought that invaded my mind.

Every day I cried uncontrollably in the restroom on my job. I cried going to and from work and walking from the bus. Suicidal thoughts flooded my mind; I even had thoughts of killing the kids. At least it would set us free, but the most dominant thought was, "How could I kill him before he killed me?" But thanks be to God (whom I didn't know); He made a way of escape for me. As fearful as I was, I made up my mind that I would get out of this mess, even if I had to die. Desperate for change, I got a divorce. I know that if I had stayed in the relationship one of us would have gotten hurt, if not killed.

Not many women in the early 1960s, at age 19, took a drastic step such as divorce, especially with three children (I had another child the year we were married, who died at one year old). I totally attribute my desire, will, motivation and determination to get out of this marriage to the grace and mercy of God (someone who had a greater power than I did). I also recognize that it was not God's will for me to get married then, even though I didn't serve Him at that time. I saw the signs, the abuse, the sadness and all the things that were evidence that I was making a mistake. I also know that He had a plan for abortion. What my life. Now, at 20 years old, I found myself single with three children and one was next? At least I had relief from being out of the abusive marriage, and that brought me some peace of mind.

I knew that divorce was the answer for me and I have never regretted it. Nonetheless, my friends (or should I say enemies)—**shame** and **guilt**—still followed me. My feelings of shame for not being able to make the marriage work just added to my continued list of failures (even though I knew it wasn't my fault). Often times when one thinks of self-destruction, "suicide" will immediately come to mind. Suicide wasn't something I thought about regularly, but I can see now how I was also destroying myself in other ways. *Still living but yet dying.*

As I mentioned in an earlier chapter, this is how I saw my life:

- My goals, dreams, and ideas were destroyed from within
- I was destroyed by my own thoughts. There was an inability to think of myself

> as being able to succeed or become a part of something
> - My self-esteem was batting a zero

During this time in the 60s, there were no television talk shows dealing with feelings and ways to solve things like there are today. I certainly didn't go to the library to research what I felt. I didn't even know how emotions and feelings operated in a person.

Today, as I look back over my life, I realize that those feelings of **shame** and **guilt** had engulfed me. Not only had they taken deep root but they had spread into other areas of my life.

Most of the time, we think of shame as a painful feeling of having lost other people's respect because of having done something wrong. Maybe it's because someone who is close to us or someone we are associated with has done something wrong. Or we see it as a loss of honor or respect or disgrace. Shameful is bringing shame or disgrace, not moral or decent. Psychologically, shame attacks the identity of a person. Feelings of shame causes one to feel that they are not good enough, or less than others. Shame denotes that one is inadequate; that you don't measure up, that you are a failure and will never amount to anything.

Then there's guilt. Guilt is having done a wrong or committed a crime. It is associated with something you've done. You can alleviate it by admitting it and making restitution for it. You can feel guilty about doing something and not feel shame. An example is if you get caught stealing a cookie out of the cookie jar, you might feel guilty. You say you are sorry, you get punished, and you go on. But shame says that you are a bad person for stealing the cookie; you are no good. What will others think? You'll never amount to anything.

Shame attacks your personal worth. Now as human beings, we don't usually process the feelings and emotions that we experience and then readily do something about them. Rather, we allow our feelings or emotions to rule, dictate and control us.

Now you can understand better that the feelings of **shame** and **guilt** that I experienced from having a child out of wedlock and from the abortions were ruling my very being. Most of the decisions I made were centered around **shame** and **guilt**.

Please understand that I did not go about saying, "Oh, I feel so awful. I'm a bad person; I'm not good enough." In spite of that, I demonstrated on the outside (by my actions) the pain that was locked inside me. As time went on, the self-destructive behavior and feelings of self-hatred continued in both subtle and blatant ways. My behaviors were manifested in a number of negative ways, the greatest of them being promiscuity.

Promiscuity: I tried to fill the emptiness that I felt inside with numerous sexual partners.

Hatred of men: While I did not realize that I hated men (after all, my promiscuity would seem as though I loved them), my innate desire was to use them to get what I could from them.

Subconsciously, I was trying to make up for the pain men had caused me, and on the other hand, my feeling of unworthiness caused me to be hurt, humiliated and sometimes used by them.

Suicidal impulses: In retrospect, there were several times I contemplated taking my life. There were a couple of people whom I thought could do a better job raising my children instead of me. I felt like such a lousy mom. Actually, I almost signed papers to give my oldest child up for adoption. Deep down inside, I loved her and I had no intention of not keeping her. I buckled under the pressure from a married couple who seemingly had more to offer her, and who almost convinced me to let them raise her. Thank God I changed my mind the night before. Afterwards, I remember feeling so guilty and confused, unable to forgive myself for not giving them my child. They had everything I didn't: a house, car, finances and a big yard.

Aborting (things and ideas): Generally, we understand that abort means, *"not to complete,* *to cancel, cut short, stop in early stages, to terminate."*

So it was with things in my life. These descriptions also fit right into my *"just get rid of it"* mindset.

- I was quitting my good government clerical job at the Depot that I had been so excited about. I wanted to work at the Western Electric factory. The older people whom I worked with begged me to at least stay at the Depot for three years. At that time, it would have given me permanent status. I only had a few more months to go, but I couldn't see it, so I quit. This was my life at almost 21 years old.

- Western Electric was a good job, but it didn't afford the benefits or the status my government job did. Anyway, what did it matter? I quit there and went back to the Depot, but not with the same status, of course. I had lost those benefits. I made several trips back and forth between those two places of employment. This was just the beginning of many jobs I held, never staying on any job more than a year to 18 months or so. I was dedicated and a very good employee and loved people, but out of nowhere, I would decide to quit my job. Years later, even after becoming a Christian and being married and raising a family, I never stayed on a job.

I was always somewhat aware of not finishing things, but I didn't see it as a matter of concern. However, as I grew older, I realized that many opportunities seemingly had passed me by.

Currently, one of my greatest battles is still aborting. Not an actual baby, but *things, plans, ideas and projects.* Many of the ideas that I have had and aborted have become someone else's gold mine. I've had ideas for starting my own business, then several years later the same idea would be established by someone else.

On another occasion, a business had the same name that I had planned to use. On the other hand, I did actually start a business. It was enjoyable and could have been quite successful, but I never developed it to its fullest potential.

I am a project-oriented person by nature, and thrive off of making things happen.

Unfortunately, I can quit right in the middle of one project and go to another one, never completing either project. Oftentimes, it is hard to do what needs to be done *now*.

It is easier to focus on doing something else. Consequently, something is left unfinished.

Even finishing this book was difficult for me. It was actually written two years before being published. But, as usual, there were some things that led me to put off this project in favor of others.

Some of the things that have been difficult for me to complete may seem insignificant, but not to me.

For example:

- Not balancing the checkbook
- Not completing the laundry (e.g. not putting folded clothes in the drawer, if they get folded at all)
- Pushing things aside until the last minute
- Not finishing chores
- Not following eating plan or diet
- Not following through with appointments (e.g. hair, nails, doctor)

While sharing my examples with another woman, she realized that she never finishes eating her meals. She takes one to two bites of it and she is finished, yet she continually eats out, buying dinners at restaurants only to discard them later. She, too, had numerous abortions and is now starting to see how she aborts many things in her life.

Please understand that many women have had various life experiences and traumas that have led to addictive behaviors, promiscuity, low self-worth, feelings of shame, guilt, rejection, depression or fear. The list is endless, yet they never have experienced an abortion. Much of what I have described can come from traumatic experiences in our lives. However, after having an abortion, these behaviors, among others, become more intensified, and may continue until healing takes place.

When I became a Christian, it was truly a life-changing experience. Just my acceptance of Christ brought immediate transformation of certain habits, but there were some areas that didn't change right away. My feelings of guilt and shame, self-destruction and self-hatred followed along. They just manifested themselves in a more glorified way. However, I didn't recognize any of them as problems connected to abortion. The self-destruction continued. This time it was through food. When Ralph and I married, my small frame was 125 pounds, and now it was getting larger. Sometimes we exchange one additive behavior for another, totally unaware of what we're doing. Promiscuity was gone, but now eating crept in. It's difficult to see how food is harmful or destructive. After all, eating is a necessity so how can it be wrong?

Usually, when a person has an eating problem such as overeating or undisciplined eating habits, they are trying to make up for a loss of something, or trying to fill a void. Overeating, drinking, thumb sucking, and obsessively chewing gum are all oral ways people use in trying to fulfill or satisfy what's missing within. It mostly starts during childhood, but not always.

Another addiction that began with me as a child was eating vanilla ice cream and Hershey's chocolate, which started at age 9 or 10. For years I had been eating vanilla ice cream and Hershey's chocolate, totally unaware that *it ruled my life*. Actually, when I was growing up, I ate it every night as my bedtime snack. I would get a bowl and pour lots and lots of Hershey's rich chocolate over two or three dips of vanilla ice cream. Then I'd eat it slowly, stirring continuously as it blended together. I loved it!

Well, you are probably asking the big question by now—so what was wrong with that? Nothing was wrong with Hershey's chocolate and ice cream, but the way I was eating it made it wrong. That was just the beginning.

My need for vanilla ice cream and Hershey's chocolate was a daily need, although I was not aware of it. Sometimes I ate it in the morning, before I went to school.

The need continued in my adult life. No matter what kind of ice cream the family ate, I was sure to have vanilla ice cream with Hershey's chocolate, and for the most part, they did too. But not everybody did as I did. Whenever we would go out to get ice cream treats as a family, I never tried anything different. If we couldn't afford sundaes, then I would take an ice cream cone with vanilla and chocolate swirl, or a double dipped cone with one chocolate and one vanilla dip.

Unknowingly, this food regimen had become a part of me. As a housewife, some days after everyone had gone to school, I would have a bowl of ice cream with Hershey's chocolate for breakfast, during lunch, and almost always at night time before going to bed.

I never even thought of the word "addiction." However, at times I do remember feeling as though I was *sneaking* to eat. I didn't want Ralph and the kids to know that my nighttime bowl of Hershey's chocolate and ice cream was sometimes my third or fourth bowl for the day. Believe it or not, this did not stop until I was in my late 40s.

Remember, *"You'll know the truth and the truth will make you free."* After participating in a group counseling session, the counselor explained that obsessive eating usually begins in childhood while trying to cover up a pain or hurt that took place, e.g. abandonment, abuse, loneliness, etc. After the session, I immediately went home, got into prayer and asked God to show me what was in me. That's when I saw the little lonely girl with long braids, sitting in front of the TV with a huge bowl of vanilla ice cream and Hershey's chocolate; it was me.

Although I had a wonderful and caring mom and grandmother who filled my life with lots of attention and love, encouragement, regular train rides to New York with my grandmother, piano and dance lessons, and lots of support, there were still emotional things missing in my life.

When my mother was a child, her relatives raised her. Part of her life was spent in a children's home. She had no contact with her mother, nor did she know her father. She also had no brothers or sisters that she knew of. The few first cousins I had on my father's side lived out of town, so there wasn't much family interaction like visiting with family members.

We were not close to other relatives that lived in our city, and we did not socialize. I had lots of friends and was very outgoing, but I was very lonely. I never liked being alone or being an only child. Moms, no matter how much they do for you, cannot make up for what a dad can. My mother had become a widow in her early 20s. I know now that I missed having a dad.

As a little girl, my friends were vanilla ice cream and Hershey's chocolate. It somehow fulfilled what was missing each night as I watched TV. But as time went on and I became an adult, it had become my enemy. I was addicted to this delicious dessert. I had to deal with this addiction and understand its effect on me. Chocolate is full of caffeine. I now know that I had my own little "high" (an addiction) going on for years. However, I was unaware that I was trying to fill the emptiness of my life.

My eating addiction was at its peak. You can see how oral satisfaction (in my case, food) became an open door for finding ways to fill the empty void and pain on the inside. At best it was a temporary and false fix. As a result of the prayer after the counseling that night, and what was revealed to me about my need for the ice cream and chocolate, I immediately stopped eating it. I still liked it but it is not something I need. As a matter of fact, I don't really like vanilla ice cream. If I eat it, it has to be with cake or something.

Today, when I become stressed or busy, I tend to think that I need it, but that's only because it was familiar to me. Whenever we get frustrated or we get disappointed, we tend to reach back to something that we can identify with that eases the pain, or gives us gratification and satisfaction. However, it is false hope. The self-destructive behavior that was exhibited by my eating habits was destroying my body. Why would I constantly put things in my body that would harm it?

- Could I subconsciously be punishing my body for the times I had misused it (babies, abortions, men)?
- If I loved myself, why would I hurt myself?
- Was this a slow suicide, a subtle way of killing myself? Both my doctor and my counselor expressed their concerns for my being overweight in the same week.

- The weight wasn't helping. As a matter of fact, it was hindering me—my knees, joints, ankles and back were all at risk.

These were just some of the ways I began to see how the abortions were affecting my life.

In the next chapter you'll find a list that may be helpful for you to identify some of the key symptoms that may result from having an abortion.

8

It Will All Be Over In The Mourning

God who comforts us in our tribulation…
2 Corinthians 1:3-4

Of all the chapters in this book, this is the one that I pray will penetrate the very soul of the women who read it.

It is especially for women who feel that there are no ill effects or problems from having abortions. I can so easily identify with you. I was on that road for so long—too long.

When thinking about why it took me so long to *"get it,"* I realized that "To Everything there is a Season" (Ecclesiastes 3:1-8).

Years ago, abortion, like many other things such as homosexuality, children out of wedlock, adultery, same sex marriages, and living in common-law, were considered to be immoral. Today, abortions are legal and widely accepted. To get an abortion is almost as common as getting a tooth pulled. Abortion clinics are in every major city. Advances in medical technology have eliminated some of the physical distress of having an abortion. This leaves many women thinking that having an abortion is a piece of cake.

Because abortions are an alternative method of birth control, and because people like having choices, countless numbers of women experience them daily. When something is so accepted by society, it becomes difficult for people to see anything wrong with it, or they override their true feelings to be a part of the "in crowd." I can see now that time was a major factor in order for me to know and tell my story of abortions.

I believe that my healing process took so long because God allowed me to walk through it so that I could teach others. Please understand—I could have learned sooner, but God doesn't override our will. In my stubborn self-will (although I kept crying out for God to free me), I felt a satisfaction and a sense of pleasure in feeling comfortable with my abortion decisions. After all, it was what I wanted, so it really didn't matter how God felt about it. Actually, I had never asked God how He felt. I just told Him that I wanted to be healed. You know the old cliché, *"what you don't know won't hurt you."* Truly, until the writing of this book, I was not at all interested in how God felt about abortions.

To be honest, I never even read much information to help me on abortions (I purposely avoided it); I didn't care. However, at various times I would try to get in touch with it (how God felt) because I knew my heart wasn't right.

But God... He and only He could see beyond that hardened, hurt heart and hear my true cry. I could see that I was limited within myself and I could go no further than where I was healed. After many of my speaking engagements, people would ask me "Where is your book? You should write a book." Although I had attempted to write for a very short period, I know now that the timing is right. I knew that what God had spoken to me, "This is your first book," would come to pass. *Most of my healing came through writing this book.*

There are various roads that we must travel before we reach a destination. I like to think of my life as "traveling down the scenic route." Each new road had something different to offer. As I look back over the roads that I've traveled, some were good. I went the right way. But I also see that there were some road signs that I did not follow. **Stop! Caution! Look Ahead! Yield!** and **Do Not Enter!**

Those roads took me the wrong way. I believe that God was always on the road with me. He was waiting for me to make a U-turn. Once I made it, I took heed and tried to follow the right road and make the right choices. On the road back, I had to do the hardest thing ever in my spiritual life. I had to *give up my will* and *what seemed right to me* concerning abortions, and let God's Word and will be settled and final. It didn't matter whether I agreed or believed the scriptures or not. I still had to give up my will.

I knew that the abortions had killed the unborn babies and *I knew that I had killed the babies* because I had given permission for the abortions to take place. There was no nice way to put it! Whether the baby was one week old or 4-½ months, life had taken place.

Even medical reports and doctors who weren't Christians said that abortion was murder, and God's word was final above all. Also, *I had to give God permission to go deep down within me* (my inward parts, and He did) and help me to see what I could not see. That's because I really wanted to serve Him.

In today's society, with abortions running rampant, many women are not prepared for the end results after the abortion has taken place. As a matter of fact, they are not even aware of what might happen later.

The main focus here is "not being pregnant." So thoughts of spiritual, physical, psychological, or social trauma (which come up later in life) that stem from having abortions are seldom considered.

Unfortunately, at the time of the abortion, the most important thing in a woman's mind is to seize the moment and do what needs to be done about the baby (that is, to abort it).

While pondering over my abortions and others who have shared their experiences with me, the revelation of these terms began to help me understand *my own self* in dealing with the abortion process. The terms associated with these emotions are **Mourning, Early Mourning** and **Delayed Mourning**.

Mourning

In general, we understand that mourning means to feel or express sorrow or grief over misfortune, loss or anything regretted.

Early Mourning

In early mourning, you experience and recognize relief, for you are no longer pregnant. In addition, you also may acknowledge the pain, sadness, sorrow, guilt, shame and other emotions that immediately followed the abortion. You don't just stop at the relief stage and this is good, especially if you follow through with abortion counseling, self-help books, or a group dealing with abortions. But if you do not, and most women won't, several things may happen.

First of all, you may dismiss what you feel by not getting in touch with that emotion. After all, it's over now and life goes on. Or perhaps your friends, co-workers, family members or others will validate your experience and how you are doing after your abortion. Unfortunately, many women get to this point. They know something is unsettled within but, after all, it's easier to move on. *At this point, this becomes delayed mourning.*

But my prayer is that:

1. You will realize that there is more, lots more. It's only just begun. You don't just stop at the **relief stage,** but you must get in touch with the other emotions as well. If you do, you will save yourself from the various effects having an abortion has later on in life. Also, you will at least begin to recognize them and get abortion counseling. Or...

2. **Get in a support group** so you can grieve properly.

DELAYED MOURNING

This is what I hope you will come out of today and realize that the relief you felt was great (I agree with you), but you can't stop there. That wasn't the end.

Abortions have deep roots and they spread. When something is delayed, it is put off, or held back. When something is not dealt with it doesn't go away, it just finds another place to harbor and grow. Your behaviors, actions, attitudes and mindsets are indicative of the abortions that you thought would go away in time.

The Grieving Process

The grieving process is in no way limited to having abortions. Whenever there is a loss in one's life, the grief process kicks in, whether we realize it or not. Actually, the grieving process must take place before a person can accept a loss. There are five stages in the grieving process. They are Shock/Denial, Anger, Bargaining, Depression, and Acceptance.

I've attended and taught workshops on dealing with the losses such as death of a loved one, sexual abuse, divorce, employment, relationships, and rape.

I mentioned abortions as a loss but I know that I was limited in my insight because of the issues that still surround my own abortions, which I couldn't figure out. I rarely read anything about abortions because I did not think it was necessary. It amazes me how I was able to avoid information on Post Abortion Syndrome (PAS).

Post-Abortion Syndrome is a set of psychological patterns that occur after the abortion. PAS appears to be a type of denial that can last five to ten years beore emotional difficulties surface. In other words, this process does not even begin until several years after the abortion has taken place. This is definitely what happened to me.

Because I never read or dealt with any abortion counseling, I didn't know there was yet another stage that precedes the first five stages. And that was the one stage I was stuck in for years—relief. I did not really know or understand that relief was a part of the healing process. However, my personal belief is that if a woman is informed of what abortion is or what should happen, it doesn't have to take that long.

Support and therapy groups for women who've had abortions will definitely help them to identify and get in touch with their feelings and grief. I believe also that as a start, the things that I am sharing in this book will give you insight and keep you from being ignorant.

THE RELIEF STAGE

The Relief Stage is the first stage you experience after the abortion.

- The abortions brought me relief. It was a way out, a type of freedom. Because the relief was so gratifying and an answer to a need (*"not another baby"*), it superseded any other emotion or pain that needed to be dealt with (or so I thought).

- Many women who abort feel exactly the way I did—relieved—not knowing that it was normal after an abortion. But they are not aware of the fact that there is more— that's just the first step.

- At the time of the abortion, many women have good reasons for their decision. All the reasons for needing an abortion seem right (as wrong as they might seem now— they were right at that time).

- The anxiety of having to carry a baby for nine months was over.

- The uncertainly of not knowing what the future holds for this unwanted child was now gone.

- There was gratefulness to God (even though I didn't know Him personally) that I made it through. I was alive and no lon- ger pregnant.

- In my emotions (feelings), there was no was no sadness, sorrow, remorse or guilt.

- In my emotions (feelings), there was no sadness, sorrow, remorse, or guilt. Because I did not experience those emotions, I thought that I didn't feel anything. What I did not understand was that relief was a natural, normal way to feel after an abortion. Obviously, for a woman who did not plan or purpose an abortion or miscarriage, her feelings would be more guilt-laden, because she wasn't really sure whether or not she did something that might have prevented it. But, for a woman who makes a decision to abort her child she normally feels relief.

- Once the relief has subsided and life goes on, it does not negate the fact that a loss has taken place in her body, and this loss needs to be dealt with.

All losses—large or small—need to be acknowledged and dealt with. This can be very hard for the woman because often times, she has not accepted the fact that she is responsible for the death of her child.

Like myself, I never even considered the meaning of "death and murder."

SHOCK OR DENIAL

When one first hears of a death of someone or when something traumatic happens, the first stage expressed is one of shock. "Oh, it's not true, they could not be dead," or "That couldn't have happened." Often the person lives in a state of denial, hoping that whatever happened is not true, or that it will go away.

With abortions, after the relief stage has sub-sided, the denial stage enters in. Some results of this stage include:

- It may be hard to remember the actual experience (you don't really like to think about it).

- You use comfortable terms to justify what you really did (e.g. I found it very difficult to say "kill" or "murder." Others may use such terms as "medically-aborted," or such terms as "medically aborted," or "terminated a pregnancy").

- It becomes easy to deny what really happened because it can be justified based on the circumstances of why you had to abort the baby.

- It's easy to deny because it's so well accepted by society, friends and doctors. After all, how can abortion be wrong when it's legal? And besides, it's your body.

- That part of my life is over. It happened years ago, so why bring it up now? The fact is that it is not over—only buried, hidden or repressed—but not over.

Remember, anything that is unresolved will come back in some form sooner or later.

ANGER STAGE

In talking with various women (and in my own life), I realized that anger can so easily be repressed, suppressed or displaced. Often times we appear to be angry about one thing, but in reality, we are angry about something else. Women are angry because:

- People they talk with (friends, relatives) felt that abortion was the best alternative for them.
- Parents, relatives or partners put pressure on them to have an abortion.
- For various reasons the fathers:
    - Did not use protection
    - Were unsupportive physically, financially and emotionally
    - Have other children and are not being responsible for your child's care
- She made the decision to abort.
- She did not have a clear understanding of the abortion procedures and the after-effects.

- God allowed her to get pregnant.
- Other women in adverse situations chose to keep their babies.

In Chapter 4 (God Has a Plan in Spite Of...), I mentioned various ways in which my anger was triggered long after my abortions took place. Anger is both good and bad. The scripture gives us permission to be angry, but not to sin because of it (see Ephesians 4:26).

Anger can be quite positive in bringing about a change. However, if not handled properly, anger will be expressed in many negative ways.

Once the anger is dealt with and worked through, forgiveness can take place and you can move on. This is a process and should be dealt with by a professional or trained abortion counselor.

Too often abortion leads to negative behaviors and then sin becomes prevalent in a person's life. For many women, one abortion leads them to three or four others.

Bargaining

Bargaining is another part of the grief process that takes place. Bargaining goes on in our minds to help us buy time to accept the truth of the situation. It becomes the "whys" and "ifs" of the matter, and other painful questions that help us face our reality.

- What if I hadn't aborted the baby?
- What if there was some other choice I could have made?
- What would the baby have looked like?
- Would he or she be a leader or someone great?
- If the father hadn't been messed up, would I have kept the baby?
- If everyone had not agreed, would I still have aborted the baby?
- If things had been better financially, would I have kept the baby?
- The baby was probably not developed enough, so does it really matter?
- What name would I have given my baby?

Even though you don't have answers for all the questions that come to your mind, it is okay to let them naturally surface and think about them, rather than deny and repress your emotions and feelings. Even though you can't bring the baby back to life, there are some ways that will help you deal with your loss. Many times, healing comes with thinking something through and coming up with a solution or an answer, rather than totally avoiding it. We will discuss some solutions further in this chapter.

Depression and/or Guilt

In most instances, when a loss takes place, there are several ways to grieve or even say goodbye. Whenever a death occurs, there are funerals; when separation occurs, there's divorce. When a woman has a miscarriage, it's okay to feel sad. But with abortion, there is no real way to know or understand how to mourn or grieve for a baby that you deliberately got rid of. Often, depression comes as a natural part of grieving.

During this time such thoughts as these may come to mind:

- I should have given my baby a chance.
- Why didn't I have it and give it up for adoption?
- What if I can never have another child?
- What if my next baby is deformed?

When processed properly, the depression stage will help women to release the anger toward themselves and others. Post-abortion counseling can help in dealing with this.

Shame and Guilt would say to you, "How could you mourn something you could have avoided?" *But the truth is that mourning brings about healing.* You should remember that any loss must be grieved. There must be some form of finality or closure, or it will remain unresolved.

DEPRESSION

I recognize now, years later, that promiscuity, overeating, and thoughts of suicide were always there. Although I wasn't aware of it, I was trying to ease the pain of the guilt I felt. The fact is that I had murdered my babies brought about feelings of guilt, shame, pain, self-pity, and self-condemnation. I can even remember dating a guy who pointed out to me how much I condemned myself. People often see in us what we can't see in ourselves.

Because most relationships are not honest and open, we don't confront one another with things that would help us. Now I know that until these emotions are acknowledged and processed, there is no real grief that can take place. I believe that if I had known what to expect and was in touch with the feelings that I repressed, I would have recognized that many of my behaviors were abortion related.

Perhaps these emotions would not have continued to rule my life for such a long period of time. It was through sexual abuse classes that I became aware of the terrible effects of abortion. However, over 30 years had passed from then to now.

**Ladies, please don't wait that long.
You can help yourself now!**

ACCEPTANCE

The Acceptance Stage cannot take place until all the other stages have been processed. A woman may think she has accepted what she did and has gone on with her life, but *true acceptance* has not taken place. What happens is the grief just gets covered up. Bits and pieces of the grief may surface from time to time, but because of the lack of understanding, it is not properly dealt with.

You may have quick, fleeting feelings and other thoughts of wondering about the baby you would have had, but as fast as you think or feel it, you also dismiss it. This is false acceptance. Again, until the actual feelings and thoughts are processed, there is no true acceptance.

Please understand that the mourning and grieving stages can be like an emotional roller coaster. One day you think you are fine, and a commercial comes on TV, or a baby appears, and you may find yourself getting angry all over again. To repeat myself, acceptance can only come when a woman has acknowledged and again dealt with all the emotions that go with grieving.

There are several things that should take place in your acceptance stage. I'll discuss two of them here.

Forgiveness. The first thing should be *forgiveness*. When we hurt, everything in us hurts, and often times we want to get even, or hurt others back. We cannot afford to hold on to feelings of unforgiveness. The scripture teaches us that we must forgive to be forgiven.

You'll have to *forgive yourself* and *anyone else* who was somehow involved in your abortion. This could be the father or the person who assisted you. The enemy of your soul would like to keep you focused on the guilt, shame, anger, relief, or other emotions that keep you bound. Many women gloat or boast in the fact that they had an abortion, refusing to acknowledge the wrong in it. That is certainly a trick of the enemy, for God desires truth in the inner man.

When you truly forgive yourself, you can stop punishing yourself by overeating, hating yourself, living in promiscuity, backbiting, and many other ways.

Read the following scriptures in the Bible that speak on the subject of forgiveness:

> Matthew 6:14-15
> 2 Corinthians 2:5-11
> Hebrews 13: 14-15
> James 5:15-16
> Ephesians 4:26-27

Letting Go. The second feature of the acceptance stage is *letting go*. There are various things that will help you to let go. Each woman may or may not need to experience letting go in the same way. Are you still asking yourself questions such as:

- Was it really a baby? If it was really a baby, where is it now?

- Will I see my baby in heaven? If so, will it know me?
- What would I have named it?

These questions can possibly be settled with Post-Abortion Syndrome counseling. For now, you may find some comfort in knowing that your unborn baby is not responsible for your choice, and it will be with the Lord.

Naming the Unborn Child

Some women find a great emotional release in naming their unborn baby, although you may not really know whether it was a boy or a girl. This brings comfort and release for some women. It's like bringing closure to what happened.

Personally, I did not see the necessity of saying goodbye to my aborted babies. However, something strange happened to me. A friend of mine happened to go to an abortion workshop. The participants were asked to name the unborn children they had aborted, and if they had not aborted any, to do it for someone whom they knew had aborted children. My friend said she immediately thought of me. Next, she began to cry profusely as she called out the names of the four boys and one girl I had aborted.

My friend told me this was an intense and traumatic time for her as she experienced my pain. I wanted to be upset with her, but I realized several things. God had caused her to stand in the gap for me, and I had always believed that the babies I aborted were mostly boys. Also, she was not aware of the fact that I had five abortions. It was truly a spiritual experience as she shared this with me.

WRITING TO YOUR UNBORN CHILD

Writing a letter to your aborted child can also help to release the things that you want to say. In a therapy session with a counselor, you can verbally release things you would like to have said. If you have a really strong relationship with God, you can tell Him what you would like to say to your baby. You should start off with statements such as:

- Something that I have always wanted to say to you is...
- If you had been here with me, I would have...
- I'm sorry I took your life.
- When I see you in heaven...

Some may want to do something in memory of their child. For instance, you could write a poem or frame a special scripture in their honor. Use your own creativity to express your thoughts to your unborn child.

True Acceptance

Note the various scenarios that can help you gain true acceptance:

- When you are able to acknowledge that you ended your unborn child's life.
- When you have expressed your emotions and grief without being controlled by your emotions.
- Knowing that God has forgiven you and you have forgiven yourself and others.

- You are no longer in bondage to guilt, shame or relief. Remember, the feeling of relief will be a form of bondage until you acknowledge your sin before God.
- When you can help others to understand the effects of abortion.
- Being able to say, by the grace of God, that you can go on, no longer living in denial, but living in the freedom that only Christ can bring.
- Realizing that God is not going to keep you from having more children (hopefully you'll be in a marital relationship for your next pregnancy); or cause you to have a deformed child because of the sin of your past.

BEHAVIORS, SYMPTOMS AND EXPERIENCES

The following list is compiled of various behaviors, symptoms, and experiences of my own and other women who have experienced abortions. At the time of this compilation, none of the women had received counseling since their abortion, but they were aware of some issues.

Physical Behaviors

- Feeling a sense of being lost or alone
- Crying when you're alone
- You can't really tell anyone the truth (How could they understand?)
- Telling everyone (Trying to find acceptance.)
- Feeling like parts of your body are missing from within

Some Fears

- Touching babies
- Never having a normal pregnancy
- You will be punished by God
- You won't be able to give birth again
- You will harm other children
- You will hate other children
- You will become jealous if someone close to you is pregnant

- Becoming pregnant and feeling that you need another abortion
- Trusting again
- Making decisions
- Being pretty or feminine

OTHERS

- Eating Disorders
- Hatred or abusive of children
- No pleasure in sex
- Turning to females for comfort and love (lesbian relationships)
- Promiscuity
- Addictions—drugs or alcohol
- Self-abuse
- Self-hatred and condemnation
- Hatred of men
- Suicidal thoughts or impulses
- Reactions on the date the abortion took place
- Unforgiveness of self and others
- Flashbacks
- Guilt and/or shame
- Depression

- Hardness of heart
- Withdrawal
- Isolation
- Sorrow and/or grief
- Remorse
- Despair
- Hopelessness
- Regret
- Anger and/or rage
- Defensiveness
- Never really dealing with anything
    - Laughing when things aren't funny
    - Won't get too serious
    - Jokes more than is necessary
    - Condemns other people
    - Fault-finding and critical of others
    - Never satisfied with self

- Afraid of intimacy
- Afraid to fully give of your self in a marital relationship
- Nightmares or fantasies about babies
- Can't stand baby showers, baby clothes, or anything to do with babies

EXPERIENCES

At a conference in which I talked briefly on abortion, I was surprised at how many women wanted to talk to me afterwards about their abortion experiences. Some of the comments they made were:

- A woman told me she finally realized that she kept having children trying to make up for the abortions she had. At that time she had seven children. Although there were marital problems, there was a need to keep giving birth.
- Another lady realized she was always surrounding herself with kids because she was trying to make up for a void within her from having an abortion.
- Women have shared that they felt guilty being nice to their children when they knew that they got rid of one. (This is actually an issue of shame—feeling you are not good enough or don't deserve to be a mom).

- One woman just happened to think about the abortion one day 15 years later. She said she began to cry from thinking about how old the child would be, and what he/she would have been like.
- Another lady had her tubes tied at a young age so she would not get pregnant again after a series of abortions, which she later regretted.

These are just some of the ways you may be affected. Remember, praying for God's guidance, Post-Abortion Syndrome counseling, and reading Christian self-help books will all help you understand the abortion process.

REMEMBER:

God has a plan for your life. Look up and move on. Don't be deceived any longer, but be relieved by knowing the truth.

9

SINS OF THE PARENTS

(YOU BETTER BREAK THAT GENERATIONAL TIE)

...visiting the iniquity of the Fathers upon the
children and the children's children unto
the third and fourth generation.
Exodus 34:7

With all the things my counselor and I discussed, it would seem that we covered everything concerning my abortions. However, there was still another *issue* (a BIG one). In our sessions, I disclosed how difficult it was for me not to tell my daughters my true views on abortion. My girls and I were very close, and we discussed all sorts of things. Whenever my daughters would confer with me about abortion, I would give them my famous script, "You know your dad's and my view on abortion, and you know what the Bible says." I always wondered if they could really tell how I felt, but they didn't express it. After all, I was Mama. I further exposed to my counselor that I knew my daughters had experienced abortions and they had on occasion asked my opinion. And, of course, I gave my usual script line, but I felt they knew I wasn't telling the whole truth.

Part of the truth was I really didn't want them experiencing abortions. I knew it was not right, but at the same time, I knew that another baby would interfere with their lives. And although I never said it to them, the thought would occur. **Just get rid of it**—you're probably not that many months along.

Be assured, I'm not happy about my thoughts, but remember the root had already grown. It was actually controlling my thoughts and actions. Just like the Bible says, a root of bitterness in you springs up and will defile many (Hebrews 12:15 NLT).

"Just get rid of it" were bitter and poisonous words. It was at this time my counselor brought to light another revelation, one that I did not expect. This was **the big one!** Here's what she said, "Susan, not only did you abort babies, but your daughters are now carrying on the generation sins of abortion passed down by you." Whoa! What a rude awakening. I suddenly felt numb. I certainly did not have to be convinced—I could see the pattern. No, I never assisted them financially in getting an abortion, but neither did I try very hard to convince them not to. If I knew in advance I just avoided it. Most of the time I was not told until afterwards, or when I overheard them discussing abortions.

Sometimes I could discern it and ask if they were pregnant. Either way, I didn't offer much advice. They knew I didn't approve, or at least they thought they did. Actually, what mother really wants her daughters having abortions? But nonetheless, I knew they would be relieved. After all, I had always been relieved.

To be confronted with the fact that my daughters had now picked up where I had left off was not at all comforting, but it was the truth. How could this have happened? How could something I did go so far? I was in my teens and early twenties when I had the abortions. That was more than 30 years ago.

All of a sudden I felt trapped. How could I get out of this? Some folks say the truth hurts. It does, but it also makes you free.

As time went on I began to mull over this new revelation. What a mess! Now I had a new title; it was certainly not one to be proud of. I could just see me at a conference being announced: "Our speaker today is Susan Ridley. who is a pastor, evangelist and abortion queen. Please greet her with 'Praise the Lord.'"

I believe that God gives you a humorous or a funny thought sometimes to help ease the real pain. I could picture this very staunch, old self-righteous, condemning women trying to keep their composure as I was announced as the speaker of the hour.

Immediately, after I finished laughing and the picture vanished, I began to cry and thank God. He had used me so mightily to help others, even with all my mess. I was still the Queen—His Woman. **He just had some more work to do on me—a lot more.**

Perhaps you're one who might not believe or have ever considered that we pass various curses, patterns, sins, and habits (some good and some bad) from generation to generation. You may know families where you see generations of alcoholism, abuse, poverty, divorce, certain fears, greed, secretiveness, abortions, selfishness, and lying, only to mention a few. It could have started with great, great-grandparents and continued on.

The Bible speaks of curses passed down to the third and fourth generations. Exodus 34:7 states, *"Visiting the iniquity of the fathers upon the children, and upon the children's children."* Particular family members are not the only ones affected by the dreadful results of generational sin. Children suffer much for the sins of their parents.

I have no formula for stopping generational sins, but there are many Christian books that can perhaps go into the subject with more detail.

In the meantime, you can take any of the following actions regardless of the generational sin:

1. Come out of denial; call sin what it is.
2. Expose it. Stop pretending that the sin does not exist.
3. Break the secret. Look at its roots; look at where it started and how far it has spread.
4. Talk about it. Don't let the enemy continually destroy you and your descendants.
5. Do something. That's exactly what I had to do. I went to Christian counseling in order to be able to get help and deal with my sin.

6. Renounce the curse or sins of the past. Renounce means "to give up a claim, belief or right; to refuse to have anything more to do with; to disown."

I wondered how many women in my parents' generation had abortions, and if so, who before me had them. I also knew that was something I would never find out, and anyway, what difference did it make? With me heading up my generation, that was enough.

As I discussed with my daughters about abortions and writing this book, they realized the fact that their experiences of having abortions would have to be exposed.

With my four daughters and myself, we had experienced over 20 abortions. Mine were done in the '60s, and theirs were done in the '90s. We were all surprised to find out that it had been so many. Just as I had expected, most of my daughters, along with many other women I talked with, had put their abortions on the back burner, not realizing or knowing it's effects. I wish I could say that the spirit of "getting rid of babies" wasn't passed on, but unfortunately it was.

My daughters and I are talking more openly about their abortion experiences, and they realize their need for healing. Because I finally began working on mine, coupled with the writing of this book, I will be able to help them. They are all Christians now and they all have children. We minister together as a mother/daughter team. As a family, we must pull together so that our daughters and granddaughters will not repeat our pattern.

I took action. If the sin of abortion runs in your generations, you can take action today. I sincerely hope that my story has helped you in some way, and my prayer is that you will pass it on.

Meet Susan J. Ridley

Susan J. (Fulton) Ridley was raised in Columbus, Ohio. Her roots began in the housing community known as Poindexter Village. She attended three Columbus schools: Mt. Vernon Elementary School, Champion Jr. High, and East High School.

Susan is a kaleidoscope of talent. She is a wife, mother, grandmother and great-grandmother—both naturally and spiritually. She is a minister, author, playwright and speaker. She has been involved in ministry for more than 50 years. Susan has been instrumental in shaping and transforming the lives of innumerable women through various community and ministry endeavors.

Susan J. Ridley

Susan and Ralph, her husband of 51 years, have been actively involved in outreach ministry all of their married lives. They are the proud parents of 5 married children, 17 grandchildren and 20 great-grandchildren, with more to come.

How to Contact Susan J. Ridley

Contact Susan at
ridleymktplace@yahoo.com